Addiction Is An Illness
We All Share

Addiction Is An Illness We All Share

Dr. Merav Nagel

Editor: Nicole Fisher

To order additional copies of this book, contact:
Xlibris Corporation
1-888-795-4274
www.Xlibris.com
Orders@Xlibris.com
127574

*This book would not be accomplished
without the support of Dr. Ralph Bradley.
Thank you Ralph for everything!*

Contents

Introduction

What is Addiction?

ADDICTION IS DEFINED as a persistent, compulsive dependence on a behavior or substance. The term has been partially replaced by the word *dependence* and substance abuse now also includes mood altering behaviors or activities. Some researchers refer to two types of addiction: 1) substance addiction such as alcoholism, drug abuse, and smoking, and 2) process addiction such as gambling, spending, shopping, eating and sexual activity. The social cost for either of these is substantial. Property crime increased 8.6% and violent crime increased 12.6% due to gambling alone.[1] There is a growing recognition that many addicts are those who are poly-drug abusers—individuals who are addicted to more than one substance or process. Addiction is a disease which can be treated with medications, counseling and support from family and friends.

Addiction is not something that is easily tested for and test results cannot be the sole basis for treatment and decisions-making. Very often patients are the last ones to make any decisions about their own health, such as taking control and responsibility for what they put in their bodies. They may not be true and honest with themselves because they are afraid of the consequences and would rather not take responsibility, accountability, and learn from it. Deception may be second

---

[1] *Deseret News*, September 2, 2012.

nature to them and a survival mechanism, much like using lies to hide and cover the unpleasant truth. The problem is that one lie creates and leads to another lie.

The Overabundance of Drugs

In the era of a "pill for every ill" there are abundant drugs and if we do not like what we take, it can be quickly replaced with another drug. Why make the effort to change our lifestyle if swallowing a pill can resolve the problem in a matter of seconds? Pharmacological companies will not go out of business, but they do not consider what drugs do to consumers in the long run. Does the problem we take that pill for really vanish for good? Does the drug guarantee that we will not have another problem in the future? Taking one drug may cause addiction to another drug as we become dependent on the first. There is a danger of taking a pill of unknown origin, which could contain any substance, even a lethal one. Most addictions are life-long disease, which means that to avoid a relapse, a person must remain sober for life. Often making adjustments or modifications to the environment, behaviors, and lifestyle is a much better solution. Many illnesses are a result of a psychosomatic cause and the root of the problem does not disappear with the best drug. Numerous medications and substances can produce false-positive or false-negative results.

Too many people rely on medications to resolve their addiction and to treat drug abuse. A new vaccine that prevents nicotine addiction does so by triggering the production of antibodies that bind nicotine in the blood and keeps it from reaching the brain. Another investigational medication is designed to induce the body's natural defenses to deactivate cocaine before it reaches the brain. Most of these medications are tested on laboratory animals. It seems to be unethical to administer street drugs to animals, but researchers claim the benefits outweigh the cost, and save human lives. Animal studies determine whether substances have addictive properties. They also guide the development of new treatments and medicines and provide key information about how they produce their curing or addictive properties.

Mental and Medical Health

Though the number of adults smoking in the US has decreased overall, 68% of those who are smoking said they are addicted.[2] According to *Brain the in News*[3], those who suffer from mental health are more than twice as likely to smoke cigarettes and more than 50 percent more likely to be obese compared to the rest

[2] *Deseret News*, September 16, 2012.
[3] *Brain in the News*, October 2011.

of the population. Heart disease, diabetes, or other physical medical conditions are often major illnesses and compound onto the problems caused by drug addiction. For those who had a heart attack, experiencing depression increases their risk for cardiac-related death three-fold. People with diabetes have double the risk of depression. Severe chronic traumatic encephalopathy (CTE) which is a progressive damage to the brain associated with repeated blows to the head has also been identified as a major cause of depression and dementia.[4] Due to the dangers of CTE amongst football players, the National Football League has launched a mental health hotline developed and operated with the assistance of specialists in suicide prevention derived from depression.

Models of Addiction

Due to the illusion that drugs could give love it was thought that abstinence required spiritual and mental context, which drew some to non-traditional models of curing addiction rather than pharmacological intervention. While the wealthy could afford treatment, others reached to substances, such as methadone, to cease tolerance and relieve their cravings. Methadone intervention helped cut criminal activity, death and HIV and healing seems to improve with heroin addicts.

Addiction used to be categorized as an "army disorder", due to the record consumption of cocaine, marijuana, and heroin after the wars. The term cross-addiction was developed and refers to dependence where, as a result of primary addiction, an individual develops a secondary addiction. This was very likely to be presented in cocaine users with alcohol, in alcohol users with marijuana, in heroine users with caffeine or nicotine. All of these addicts are affected by the pleasure part of the brain, the mid brain, the limbic system, which all take part in the dopamine hypothesis. Most crime and violence were found to occur in the context of drugs and alcohol abuse. In order to fix the problem psycho-stimulants were frequently prescribed in addition to a group therapy.

According to Alcoholics Anonymous, those who were addicted stayed addicted due to chemical disease and imbalance in the brain. The disease model implies that the cause, origin, and symptoms are a defect which cannot be changed. Therefore, those who are at risk of relapse will probably be reusing drugs if preventive measurements are not taken.

The basis of the harm reduction model, which was to reduce the harm of unsafe drugs with the main concern being that the individual stayed alive, became controversial. The problem with this model was that patients did not need to come ready to change and abstinence was not a requirement. Nicotine consumption was also on the rise during this time. Physicians offered nicotine gums as part of the

---

4   *Deseret News*, August 5, 2012.

harm reduction model to eliminate smoking. At high doses, however, benefits did not meet. Later it was reported that nicotine gums delivered more nicotine to the blood stream.

Therapeutic communities are often a preferred model to the harm reduction model. This is a type of group therapy where every resident has a job: they work in the kitchen, serve, clean, paint and repair; they run the offices to assist professionals who provide medical care, legal services, classroom instructions, and vocational counseling. Members act as staff aids and deputies. They are part of treatment and take a responsibility for its success. Good performance and attitude are rewarded and reinforced with promotions. Poor performance and violations of house regulations are punished. At the top of the hierarchy are members who are former drug abusers themselves, graduated the program and have been trained in the clinical methods. Their experience allows them to relate easily to the experiences of new residents. They function as role models; they encourage self-examination that leads to understanding responsibilities and change. The longer one remains in the community therapy, the better the chance of success and the greater the degree of psychological improvement. The therapeutic community model has many advantages, but is sometimes perceived as brainwash when the goal is not freedom from drugs, but rather allegiance to a religious or a political orthodoxy.

Faith based approaches can be seen in therapeutic communities. Gary Ryan, an inmate, wrote in his book that abusing drugs and alcohol gave him comfort for awhile, but then came the discomfort. Prison was a blessing to him because he did not have access to drugs, and the therapeutic community he was in became his awareness. Alcohol and drugs often mask and numb negative thinking and therefore the network of support groups outside of prison is a key component in reducing recidivism rates. Prison is sometimes perceived as a privilege because it provides a rehab program, free health care, food, shelter, hygiene conditions, and personal time to think, read and develop artistic hobbies (music, painting, or writing) as part of therapy.

The best interventions that are relevant to the community model are directed at risk and protective factors, which play part in the community's needs, resources and readiness to act. The cost benefit of substance abuse prevention to the community can be up to $36 in savings for every $1 invested. On average, funding for treatment cost is $10,000 for a state, $5,000 for a county, $7,500 for a city. Estimated personnel cost for one year is $16,900, it cost $16-20/hr to hire a coordinator, $6100 for training, community needs, data collection and implementation. Having health insurance can affect the type of treatment used. Employment is an enabling factor because it can provide payable access to health insurance.

The Cost of Addiction

Vast amounts of dollars have been spent on the war on drugs. The cost of illness is complex and covers three main areas of inquiry: what the connection between addiction and various adverse outcomes is (such as medical and social problems), to what degree addiction is directly responsible for its cost, and how the cost is determined.

The annual cost of substance abuse in the United States is estimated as $2.76 billion. This is part of the cost of healthcare, loss of productivity, crime, and motor vehicle accidents. Recovery and treating withdrawal symptoms call for medical and mental interventions which cost tax payer money.

Anything can be abused and can become an addiction if it is used in excess. Even prescriptions of aspirin or Tylenol contribute to healthcare cost. Although we do not become addicted to them as to other drugs prescribed for emotional and psychiatric conditions we may feel psychologically dependent on them. The Drug Abuse Warning Network has warned against fatalities caused by addiction in emergency rooms. Cost of direct healthcare is measured and estimates are made of lost productivity resulting from addiction and other costs associated with crime and accidents, in addition to the cost of medications.

Medications have been used for withdrawal from addictive drugs because withdrawal is associated with a decrease in the brain's ability to feel pleasure. Medications which have been used to treat addiction and overdose (e.g Maltrexone) reduced relapse. Methadone maintenance treatment has allowed heroin addicts to enter recovery. Among drugs which block cravings and assist in relapse are the antidepressants imipramine and fluoxetine, and the mood stabilizers carbamezepine and valproate. Contingency management is the intention to help counteract the classical conditioning when the addict was exposed to an environment where drugs were being used which resulted in cravings.

Genes play an important role in the addict's vulnerability to dependence and resilience. The addict may have had a troubled childhood, or suffered from anxiety or depression which was never treated. After years of abstinence, when the craving has been reduced to almost negligible thoughts, a small exposure to the drug is all it takes to restart the abuse and to bring back the intensity of the compelling urge that has been programmed into the brain.

Differences between Abuse and Dependence

The definitions of addictive disorder have ranged widely from a nomenclature based upon the presence or absence of physiological dependence to constructs relying on legal, social, and/or psychological problems associated with substance use. Individuals understand their own behavior and put it into a meaningful context on the basis of their culture, personal history and psychodynamics; family and other object relations; psychopathology, and other specific and nonspecific factors. Physical dependence upon a drug or upon alcohol also produces meaningful relationships between time and/or space, and subjective mood and behavior. Where heavy drinking is normative in certain societies in Europe and Russia, psychopathology appears to be a less significant risk factor for alcoholism. As marijuana use has become wide spread in the US over the past two decades, use per se is no longer limited to deviant or peripheral groups, and psychopathology has become less important as a risk factor of use by veterans.

The criteria for diagnosing abuse or dependence are based on the consequences that have occurred. The prevailing culture is an added factor. A smoker in the 1950s would have less severe addiction than a smoker today, because addiction was not a concern.

Sometimes people go through a period of abusing substances during stressful periods in their lives, but when the crisis is over there is no record of the abuse. Addiction occurs when the continued use of the substance becomes the focal point of life. When that change occurs, even when it is subtle, all other aspects of life (such as relationships, jobs, responsibilities, and goals) become less important than the drug. Incarceration or even death may result before the addict has the chance to realize the severity of the problem and enter treatment.

Addicts may be living in an abusive situation at the time that they choose to experiment and the relief that they get from painful feelings is a powerful reinforcer. The need to conform to a group may be very strong particularly for young people. Especially vulnerable are those with poor impulse control or low stress tolerance, and people who have difficulty learning from negative consequences. If they have relatives with drug dependence they are at a substantially increased risk of becoming addicted to any drug including alcohol.

Type I alcoholics tend to have mothers who are alcoholics; to have the onset of alcoholic drinking in their 30s or 40s; to be anxious, rigid, and emotionally dependent; and to experience loss of control. These alcoholics tend to engage in binge drinking. Type II alcoholics tend to have fathers who are alcoholics; to have the onset of alcoholic drinking before age 25; to have problems with conduct, aggression, and impulsiveness; and inclination for novelty-seeking behaviors. These alcoholics tend to be continuous drinkers.

Those with a genetic risk for alcoholism do not seem to have as much impairment in motor functioning when they drink the same amount of alcohol. If the family history is positive for alcoholism, there is much less body sway apparent than if the family history is negative. At a lower risk are those who lack a certain form of the enzyme alcohol dehydrogenase which breaks down acetaldehyde (for example, those of Asian descent are prone to this condition). They build up large amounts of acetaldehyde in their system, which causes them to feel ill with a flushing rapid heartbeat or burning in the stomach.

Alcoholics report high levels of craving for alcohol in those circumstances associated with dysphoric moods and may be at greater risk of relapse. There is much less need to become addicted to opiates in order to feel pleasure and numb the pain, similar to alcohol binging, when a person's family is supportive and intact. When there are opportunities to socialize and participate in rewarding activities, the pressure to use drugs or drink has less effect.

At increased risk of addiction are those who have suffered abuse or have been victims of crime, trauma, severe accidents, or natural disasters. Mood altering drugs override the brain's emotional and moral center. For instance, a link was found between Type II alcoholism and antisocial personality which overlaps with attention deficit disorders. Type II alcoholics judge their own actions by utility rather than by morality.

Addictive drugs interact in one way or another with the part of the brain known as the pleasure center. Alcoholics and their relatives have an exaggerated secretion of endorphins. Endorphins are naturally occurring opiates, and levels of beta-endorphins tend to rise in those with a family history of alcoholism. When dependence develops, the brain quickly learns that it can feel normal when the substance is present. Many people who are depressed or anxious do not have ready access to psychiatric services, and they come to feel that the use of alcohol or drugs as coping mechanisms is a useful compromise to feel normalcy and pleasure again.

The over-use of alcohol damages the muscle tissues which is most serious when the damage occurs to the heart muscle. When the heart does not pump effectively heart failure is the result. A damaged liver leads to problems with slow blood clotting factors. A hemorrhage then is very serious because the liver is not clearing wastes and a build-up of ammonia can occur in the blood stream leading to inflammation of the brain and decreased consciousness. Gastritis can cause pinpoint bleeding which can result in gastrointestinal hemorrhage. Alcohol irritates the pancreas and depletes insulin; without insulin the body cannot control blood sugar and causes a diabetic condition. Why with all these risks do they continue abusing alcohol?

Having an addictive personality is used by alcohol and drug abusers as an excuse for continuing their addictive behaviors and not taking responsibility for recovery. Biologically based brain disorders increase the risk that a person will develop addiction, and there appears to be an inherited tendency for addiction. However, it only accounts for about half the dependence, and does not correlate with any particular personality characteristics. Every major class of abused drugs interacts with the same part of the brain where most of the learning and reasoning takes place. Even drugs which are used to treat mental illness override normal systems in the brain to produce artificial mood states, and cause a rebound effect.

Confusion between abuse and dependence arises because we are limited to observing and describing behaviors when what we are trying to define involves a change in the way the brain functions. Addiction is a brain disorder that some people are more prone to develop because of genetic, psychological, or environmental risk factors. However, the distinction between abuse and dependence is not always clear.

Overmedicating and Abuse of Prescription Medications

Why do so many nurses smoke? Why do so many people age quickly and why is there so much obesity? Research indicates that the main reasons concern stress, depression and pain. The US is growing dependent on pain relief and pain relievers. People become addicted to prescription drugs they can obtain over the Internet or from a clinic (e.g. Vicodin and methadone). They may forge a medical order to obtain a prescription. Patients also do "doctor shopping" for prescription medications; they go to multiple doctors to seek relief of their pain. Some patients may steal items of value from others in order to have the money to purchase prescribed drugs or steal prescription pads. This situation is particularly painful for family members who are aware of a drug problem but do not wish to turn their relatives over to the police.

The guidelines for opioids are to be used only as directed; 83% of Oxycodone users and 15% of morphine users have died since 1998. Users are also more vulnerable of dying from prescription drugs. Methadone is more fatal than any other drug and causes about 61% annual fatal illness amongst users. There is a higher circulation of certain drugs, which contributes to more illness and death than deaths caused by motor vehicle accidents. Recent statistics also show that of the 32% of males and 46% of females who die due to complications from obesity, prescription medications were the cause of death in 28% of those individuals. The government can do much more than giving money to invent pills, and can help stop this epidemic by putting drugs through more clinical trials. The questions that should be answered through such trials are: what are the safest and most effective methods for treating pain and mental illness, how strong the pain is and how much opioids should be given?

Health care providers can do more to inform their patients of the dangers of prescription drug abuse. They should educate patients that cocktails (alcohols with opioids) can be hazardous because of the combination of depressant and anti-anxiety effects. Use of pain relievers for non-medical purposes in 2008 was related to 432 drug deaths and 268 were from prescriptions of opioids. The leading cause for usage was to relieve mental and psychological pain or psychosomatic disease. It may be impossible to be completely free of pain, but these individuals can make an agreement to take medications as prescribed. They can take medications at the lowest, effective dose and frequency needed in order to be able to function daily.

There are guidelines that need to be followed for taking opioids in conjunction with physical therapy and becoming active.

Sometimes it may be helpful to identify the population in need by race, socioeconomic status, religion, education, and geographic location for education and intervention. The likelihood for substance abuse increases with certain factors; depression, anxiety, lack of social skills, child abuse, injuries, delinquency, teen pregnancy, dropping out of school, violence, and conduct behavior. The solutions are family classes, employment, communication for improved health and well being, positive self-talk and mental health therapy. These individuals are likely to be unemployed, uninsured, substance abusers and smokers. They also do not have access to health resources and information, and ignore warning signs for illness and abuse.

The main danger is getting painkillers and using them for other reasons unrelated to pain: for instance, depression and anxiety. Misuse and abuse appear in 82% of those who suffer from chronic pain (backache, headache, and neck pain). Mental health problems appear in 49% of the diagnoses, mainly depression, but also bipolar and anxiety.

Mental and psychological pain has long been associated with physical and mental illness. However, a higher percentage of people (82%) have used pain killers for chronic pain (headache, neck pain, fibromyalgia, and arthritis), than for smoking (50%), substance abuse (49%), mental illness (49%), obesity (37%), or for stress and depression caused by their unemployment (62%). Of these individuals, 27% had no insurance. It is likely they have poor self-esteem and may be even suicidal when self-medicating.

Pain is the body's signal that something was damaged and it needs to heal. In order to heal the body has to drain toxins from a selected area, restore normal blood flow, and reduce inflammation. Since the pain is unlikely to disappear by itself, the problem requires a competent and attentive doctor. The symptoms, however, may undermine an emotional, physiological, and mental cause.

If a clinician ignores any of these impacts it may become a struggle to treat the patient. Very few physicians have specialized training in pain management and only three percent of US medical schools have been offering a separate course. In order to recoup the ability to function patients should explore non-medical and non-invasive interventions. Pills are addictive and if the individual takes enough of any of them, s/he becomes dependent. Certain drugs affect balance, judgment, memory, speech, vision, and digestive function. They may cause intense constipation, nausea, mood swings, sleep-pattern disruption and depression.

Over the counter oral pain medications contain chemicals that are harmful with dangerous side effects damaging the kidneys, liver, and other vital organs. They mask the pain as they add more toxins to the blood stream. Mental interventions are safer. For example, in guided imagery, the therapist helps patients imagine themselves in a calming place. Many patients visualize the beach or the mountains.

Guided imagery is often combined with other complimentary interventions such as movement-based therapy, nutritional and herbal remedies, mind-body energy healing, and lifestyle change. Cognitive-behavioral therapy, in which the patient describes the thought process and the therapist helps the patient learn to challenge irrational thoughts actively, is also recommended. Curing the underlining cause may resolve the problem, while a drug which promises a cure to the problem may be false.

As more young people are exposed to pills as a coping mechanism, doctors are overworked, uninterested, and under trained to deal with prescription drug abuse among their patients. Although, pain medicines have become the most commonly abused form of prescription drug (especially narcotics), other forms of prescription drugs are also abused (stimulants, diet pills, and psychiatric medications such as sedatives and anti-anxiety drugs). Prescription drug abuse may occur because individuals wish to feel euphoria, lose weight, stay awake, alleviate pain, control their stress symptoms or withdraw from the drug. Antidepressants are often used to combat the clinical depression that occurs with withdrawal. The deprivation or the withdrawal from a substance can cause the person to feel many emotions.

Certain drugs and foods release serotonin and endorphins and can enhance mood. An individual will use drugs or alcohol to cope with intolerable thoughts or emotions such as severe anxiety or depression. Unrealistic expectations are part of this, and they may feel that no matter what they do and how much they try, it will never be good enough. There is no hope, no control, and no outlet.

Developing Tolerance and Addiction

Tolerance

Physical tolerance refers to the fact that a person might think s/he wants a drink, but actually needs the drink to treat withdrawal. Biological mechanisms cannot explain relapse and there is a need for other explanations such as learning theories, or drug induced changes in the brain or a disease concept.

People who are addicted to some types of drugs require higher than normal doses of other drugs to achieve an effect. Cross tolerance to similar substances is quite common. If the abuser develops tolerance to one type of depressant drug s/he will have increased tolerance to other depressant drugs. Alteration in the function of the chemical in the brain causes the cells to be very sensitive to any kind of stimulation and when the cells are unstable it takes only little provocation to produce a reaction. Tolerance may develop to one effect of the drug and not to another.

Once tolerance to alcohol is developed, the individual becomes deficient in vitamin B-1 or thiamine which is important in processing and storing memory. When the part of the brain in charge of this function is destroyed it causes the addict to lose the capacity to retain any new information. Alcohol causes generalized damage to all nerve cells which leads to dementia or loss of intellectual functioning.

Another concern is tolerance to barbiturates which effects progress from sleep to anesthesia to respiratory depression. Withdrawal from barbiturates can be very dangerous, starting with agitation, anxiety, muscles cramps, and developing into seizures, delirium, and possibly death.

Death from overdose of opiates is frequently due to the depression of the respiratory reflex. Cravings wane over a span of 10–15 minutes provided the addict does not use the drug and diverts the attention to something else. The temporary relief the substance gives has long diminished, but stopped usage for prolonged periods of time will eventually fail. Repetitive use to avoid the symptoms of withdrawal contributes to the addiction. Tolerance is never cured but it can go into remission. Shakiness, anxiety, irritability, and sometimes psychotic reactions are seen in people who develop tolerance which is a reaction to the absence of a depressant drug. Fatigue, sleepiness, depressed mood and increased appetite are symptoms in those whose brain is reacting to the absence of stimulants.

As a higher tolerance is reached, more money is needed to fund the addiction. Addicts take away neurological funds from their own necessities, because the drug becomes a necessity of its own when the brain has learned that the drug produces pleasure. Having given addiction the first priority they divert funds to support it. The pleasure center in the brain sends signals to other parts of the brain and motivates the addict to use the substance again. Once this has occurred, the choices made about the use of drugs become more and more irrational. The addicts become more and more self-centered. When dependence is questioned, the addict defensively blames others instead of looking at him/herself. Craving for the substance may change one's life in negative ways as a result of the behavior. Addicts are more likely than others to commit violent crimes against others and family members. Prohibition of the drug leads to the growth of an underground black market and organized crime.

The Etiology of Addiction

The complex interaction of the person, the underlying dysregulation that s/he experiences, and the way an addictive substance serves to address and perpetuate the dysregulation contributes to the sustained disorder. For those who have suffered major psychological trauma, emotions are experienced in the extreme. They are either overwhelming and unbearable or numbing and confusing. Human distress and psychological suffering whether resulting from a psychiatric disorder or not, are at the root of most addictive behavior. Addictive substances and behaviors can relieve, sooth, calm, or change distress, thus giving an enormous power to dominate and take over a person's life.

The etiology of addiction continues to demonstrate learning and conditioning theory as an explanation. Learning and conditioning theory explains the etiology of addiction based on experimental studies. In a study with mice, less happy animals under restrictive conditions were apt to find addictive drugs more appealing. When patients responded to the question, "What did drugs do to you when first used" most replied that it made them feel normal and calm, or made their anger go away and allowed them to function. Some stressed the intolerable feelings of rage, hurt, shame, and loneliness that they attempted to relieve with the drug.

Given that negative emotions elicit craving, drug use allows for modulate painful affect and protects the drug from giving direct expression to these destructive impulses. Alcohol abusers present a high degree of defensiveness and use repression and denial to inhibit uncomfortable emotions. Cocaine-use disorders and depressive symptoms are common comorbid conditions often accompanied by alcohol use.

Genetics influence the development of depression and alcoholism. Identical twins have about twice the concordance rate for alcoholism (50% alikeness, 25% for maternal twins). If there was alcoholism in the family, an individual would have a three times increased risk of becoming an alcoholic. If alcoholism alone was determined by heredity factors, there would be 100% concordance rate for identical twins. It is unknown whether or not these same findings (genetic factors) hold true for susceptibility to other addictive substances (cocaine, heroin, nicotine).

Genetics indicate a possible link in addiction. Some adoption studies of children raised apart from their biological parents indicate that biological children of drug addicts are above average in becoming addicts themselves. Adopted children may be at a lower risk genetically, but are more influenced by other factors in the environment due to the fact that addiction is a self-regulation disorder, in which the addictive behavior is an attempt to correct or deal with difficulties in regulating emotions, self esteem, relationship, and self-care.

Parental neglect or abuse is not necessary for the development of substance abuse disorders. Parents, however, can and do impact their children's behavior, and they can protect them from developing such disorders.[5] In twin studies, when the first twin develops alcoholism the second twin has a 50% chance of developing alcoholism. Girls who suffer childhood sexual abuse are more likely to develop an alcohol disorder. In a violent and socially disrupted childhood a sense of well-being and inner comfort becomes elusive, leaving its victims chronically addicted and incapacitated as adults. Three social and economic areas that influence susceptibility to developing an addiction are availability, social conditions, and cultural expectations. Social and economic contexts or environments and the availability

---

[5]   Khantzian, E. J., & Albense, M. J. (2008) Understanding Addiction as Self Medication: Finding Hope Behind the Pain. Lanham, MD: Rowman & Littlefield.

of addictive substance are factors that cannot be ignored in the development of substance abuse disorders. The debilitating effects of addiction are much more severe among the poor and socially disposed. Oppressed minorities and victims of social upheaval and unrest are at higher risk for substance abuse. They exhibit character styles and behavior patterns that predispose them to addictive behavior. Poverty, unemployment, and welfare dependence are fed and fueled by addiction to drugs and alcohol. Attempts of self-medicating are self-defeating because at the end, the individual winds up with two problems–the original social and economical hardships and a secondary–the addiction.

Addiction is not only related to loss of jobs and multiple medical problems, but also to ruined relationships. It is not clear what comes first, however the addict becomes less and less concerned with the needs of others, and more and more concerned with him/herself. Addicts who are narcissists are egocentrics; they never grow out of blame, projection, and denial. They learned these defense mechanisms in childhood. Problems with drug abuse that begin in childhood do not go away in adulthood. For instance, most smokers began their habit when they were in their early teens. If the substance behavior could not be used or performed, the individual felt physically and psychologically deprived.

No matter what the drug of choice is, addiction is powerful and compromises lives. A moral deterioration occurs while the abuse is progressing in a cycle of denial, rationalization, and justification. Addicted individuals may be insensitive to the needs of others, and many develop resentment. Denial is an unconscious defense mechanism where the addict knows a lot about the particular dangers of the drug of choice but s/he cannot envision life without it. The addict feels hopeless about ever being able to stop using it, and convinces him/herself that nothing would happen if s/he continues using it. Common distortions or unrealistic thinking are false beliefs such as "I can quit any time I want to", or "I have to die somehow, might as well die happy".

Early-life abuse may cause permanent changes in the brain. The person may develop an anxiety disorder or depression that seems to be eased by alcohol or drug use. Psychosomatic symptoms may manifest as severe depression, panic disorder, hallucinations, insomnia, dread and worry. Often people who experience these symptoms take alcohol and drugs either as a temporary escape, to provide relief from their symptoms and feel normal, or as a permanent solution.

Personality characteristics, impulsivity, or sometimes psychiatric symptoms can increase the likelihood of using drugs. High energy individuals possess a magnified need for elation and excitement. Taking stimulants to accentuate the need for hypomania may be dangerous. Likewise taking sedatives, tranquilizers and opiates to calm the central nervous system (due to significant problems with emotional stability, irritability, anxiety, and depression) cause addiction and dependence. The same applies to symptomology associated with attention deficit hyperactivity disorders (ADHD).

Young people and adults with ADHD love marijuana because it helps calm and focus their attention. However, marijuana can cause psychotic symptoms such as delusions and hallucinations. Individuals with ADHD who take stimulants are as much likely to develop substance abuse disorders and nicotine dependence. In face of the significant association between nicotine dependence and depression symptomology, some researchers have tried to explain how much of the present negative behaviors of the addicted personality as a pleasure seeker or self destructive character originates from psychoanalysis. Dr. Lower Kolb proposed a psychoanalytic model of character defect that includes narcissism, dishonesty and antisocial (psychopath).

Detoxifying and Withdrawal

Addiction is a chronic, relapsing, and remitting illness. It means that an addict may relapse in the future. If detox is required more than the treatment itself, it is clear the intervention is not effective.

To detox the recovered addict must work with a physician. Patients must disclose everything pertaining to their medical conditions, and the drugs and the medications they have been using. This should be in conjunction with a drug counselor who can support the process of detoxifying and coordinate relapse-prevention. One of the hardest parts in the process may be for the addict to give up control to someone else to decide what medications he/she should put in their body. Most physicians are uneasy about working with drug addiction. Many have been betrayed by patients who lied to them in order to obtain controlled substances that they abused or by saying they lost their medications, "accidentally dropping their meds down the sink".[6]

During detoxification and withdrawal the recovered addicts will exhibit a chemically altered mood; a physiologically based compulsion to continue using; a neurologically impaired ability to make judgment; and an emotional vulnerability by responding to goodwill with anger or denial.

The terrible feeling of withdrawal, rather than the common perception of being "high", keeps many individuals with addiction continuing to use drugs. These individuals can relearn that they do not need the "quick fix" and that all problems do not need to be fixed or erased immediately by drugs.

Like alcohol and opiates, physiologically crystal meth withdrawal is not dangerous. However emotionally, crystal meth withdrawal can be debilitating and painful. The common experience of chronic users during a crash is extreme fatigue and low mood. They have difficulty experiencing pleasure, can feel depressed, and can even have suicidal thoughts. Depression can take various forms; dark mood,

---

[6]   Khantzian, E. J., & Albense, M. J. (2008, p. 109)

sadness, hopelessness, panic and anxiety. Appetite is sometimes greater and the need for sleep increases, but is irregular; it's easy to doze off in the middle of the day, while having nightmares and insomnia at night. Medications to ease psychological distress, such as benzodiazepines, are potentially addictive and abusable as much as Ativan and Valium.

Sex and crystal meth stimulate the same brain-reward pathways. The compulsive drive to use crystal meth, against all logical sense, can create a seemingly unstoppable drive to have sex. When crystal meth makes sex appealing there is always the risk of health protection (e.g. HIV). Use of crystal meth may be accompanied by high blood pressure and diabetes. Blood pressure medications have worked by blocking the release of adrenaline signals from a nucleus in the brain that can cause anxiety and distress.

A compulsion to have gratifying sex when the person is on crystal meth is a physiological state that the brain could never reach on its own. Regular sex seems pointless because after repeated and intense depletion of dopamine, recovery from damage to brain cells takes a long time. Recovered addicts must remove as many reminders of crystal sex from their lives as they can. It is the meth and the sex to which the addicts really emotionally connect with. Memories may return in flashes, but the flashes become briefer and less frequent if they do not succumb to them through relapsing. The compulsive aspect of addiction may be neurophysiologically tied to pathways stimulated by the drug.

Wellbutrin is helpful in meth recovery and may even protect some brain cells from the damage caused by the meth use. It may take several days to weeks to restore enough dopamine to improve mood, energy, memory, and clarity of thinking. However, frustration often causes the restart of meth use because it seems like the quickest and easiest way to feel better again.

Addicts will likely revert to Wellbutrin and other medications to establish a sleep/wake cycle. Sleep medications include antihistamines, because over the counter sleep aids are not strong enough. Addicts may ask for benzo-like medications, such as Ambien, Sonata, and Lunesta, which are easily abusable and cause psychotic symptoms. These medications have the same addictive potential as benzodiazepines. In addition, recovered addicts could have an accidental drug interaction that can have serious medical consequences.

After heavy and regular use of crystal meth, it may take 6 to 20 months for the brain to reach a level of functioning close to how it had worked before that individual ever used meth. The strong need for immediate gratification and a low tolerance for frustration are two psychological features that are usually present in most drug addicts. The addicts who go through detoxification and withdrawal have to ask if the drug was an option or a necessity, since it affected and threatened their entire life.

Many of the meth addict's behaviors and moods (such as lying, hiding, withdrawing, moodiness, irritability, paranoia, rageful outbursts, and depression) are a result of crystal meth highs, crashes and cravings. A care giver should have a conversation with the addict out of their compassion for the addict; the more specific the care giver can be, the less room s/he leaves for argument or denial. Reminding the addicts of their goals and desires, or how great they are when they are not using the drugs, does not leave anything for negotiation which is unhelpful. It leaves the addict to think about their progress, achievements, and future.

A caregiver shouldn't be available for emotional support if the addict starts to become emotionally (and perhaps physically) abusive to the caregiver. If the addict continues to push, manipulate, or mistreat others, and all attempts to change this have failed, then the relationship with that person should be terminated. Only when addicts start to really care about how they act, then both parties can benefit from emotional support.

Addiction is a lifelong medical illness that can be treated but not cured. There are hopes and reasonable expectations in detoxifying and going through withdrawal. If addicts continue to work hard at addressing slips back into drug use, they would gradually decrease in frequency and become easier to avoid.[7]

---

[7]   Lee, S. (2006). *Becoming Crystal Meth Addiction.* New York: Marlow & Company.

The Origin and Trafficking of Drugs

Mexico

MORE DRUGS ARE coming from Mexico, and more are coming to Mexico from China and India. Some of the Mexican methamphetamines are highly pure which means that they are far more powerful drugs than users may anticipate. Most of the illegal drugs sold from Mexico are managed by organized crime syndicates who are often violent. They are often involved in criminal trafficking of humans, especially females, who are brought to the US for prostitution. Some women prostitute themselves as an act of despair in order to obtain illegal drugs.

On April 11, 2011 it was reported that Mexico contacted authorities in search of the dozens who vanished from buses as they crossed northern Mexico headed to the US. Authorities speculated that these people were pulled of the buses and fell victims to brutal crime. In a country where the violence seems endless, the lives of more than 34,000 people were taken in the first years of the continuous, bloody drug war since President Phelipe Calderon launched his offensive against organized crime in 2006. No one knows how many people have gone missing at the hands of drug cartels. In 2011, loads of marijuana were found coming over the

US borders through Tijuana and into Arizona, with 60–70 million dollars in one single transaction.

Hardened in the street and prisons of California and deported in the 1990's to the Central American countries where they were born, the members of the Mara Salvatrucha street gang swiftly grew into a force of heavily tattooed young men carrying out kidnappings, murder and extortion. An alliance between the Maras and the most feared criminal organizations in Latin America further undermined the US-backed effort to fight violent crime and narcotics trafficking in the region. The brutal Mexican paramilitary drug cartel has seized control of large parts of rural northern Guatemala in its campaign for mastery of drug-trafficking routes from South America to the United States. The Zetas, formed more than a decade ago by defectors from Mexico's army Special Forces, have already joined the local drug kingpins in the Guatemala countryside and recruited turncoat members of Guatemala's military Special Forces for operations in Mexico. Zetas have trained a group of Maras inside Mexico. There is some evidence that other Mexican cartels have paid Central American street gangs to sell drugs for them. The war on drugs increased drug arrests, convictions, and prison sentences and is the central factor in mass incarceration. More than half of new prison sentences to state prisons between 1985 and 2000 were for drug offenses.

Ending mass incarceration due to drug related offenses would better focus investment in institutions–schools, early childhood education, drug and alcohol treatment, housing, and job programs–that are vital to America's future, and more effectively address social problems. Grounded in the views on love and forgiveness, Dr. Martin Luther King Jr. explained that systems of inequality rely on contentious blindness and indifference. There are alternatives to prisons, and we cannot be indifferent to ending mass incarceration.

In Mexico there is an organized crime (crimen organizado) where the government and the police are fully involved in promoting narcotics trafficking. A lack of morals and integrity on the part of authorities, which is evident in their actions of accepting bribes, leads to the production of more crime. In 2011, 7 mayors were reported murdered. Children drop out of schools at 2nd grade and at the age of 14 join the mafia. Children learn this is the easiest and the fastest way to make money. Children commit to crime because they have nothing else to lose. They feel there is no future if they were born into the reality that is poverty and drugs. The drug cartel may offer incentives like free cell phones, weapons, and luxuries. Children are offered $3000 for every victim's head which in 2011 brought the teen delinquency rate to 74%.

In Mexico, money "governs" the state; if you have money you can buy "justice" and you can be who you want to be. Organized crime drives the Mexican's justice system. Three judges let an assassinator, who cut and brutalized his wife, go back home. On the same day he repeated another murder by killing his wife's mother. The director of a prison helped dangerous inmates escape to the US.

The authorities have an interest to keep the status quo, keep the people ignorant and uneducated, controlled and brainwashed. The TV repeatedly plays propagandas, cheering the government. The government focuses on construction, building roads and putting more traffic signs–anything which distracts citizens from real problems. The commercials are full of aggression and sex as another tactic to distract the mind from the real core problems of this nation. Beer and coffee, as part of this culture's identity, are used as a tool to keep the people happy and quiet. Many government officials rob the people's tax money to augment their own salaries. One mayor received $50,000 a month while more the 30% of Mexican citizens lived under the poverty line. Innocent people are affected by the violence of drugs. Each day children and mothers lose their lives due to accidental killings by the traffickers. The lives of many policemen in Mexico are ended while performing their duties. It affects everyone everywhere; it spreads and proliferates like a disease.

The drug dealers offer free drugs to make their members addicts. They promise the drug will make them feel better when they feel ambivalent, anxious or guilty about committing immoral and illegal actions. Gradually, their victims lose control to the drugs and become abused and manipulated by the dealers to commit more crimes and to give away all they have to the drugs including their bodies. The most vulnerable groups for exploitation are women and children. Chauvinism keeps women submissive, dependent, and victims of abuse and acceptance. They never rebel even when it is obvious that they are in a disadvantageous situation.

The government's job is to keep teens off the street and get them engaged in learning or playing an instrument. Teaching them positive affirmation allows them to feel they are in control of the situation and can succeed. Writing about their stress boosts their brain power. Mental imagery, such as with writing, relieves stress while fast beta brain wave activities are associated with preventing relaxation. Teenagers are attracted to marijuana, alcohol, tranquilizers, and pain killers to relax. Unfortunately, scientists have been unable to explore pathways from one part of the brain to another, but they believe these pathways are the key to understanding brain-based disorders and susceptibility to drug addiction.

The adolescent brain is less able to control stress and rage, and weapons in teens' hands can be deadly. The narcotics traffickers take advantage of teens' brain immaturity in the prefrontal cortex. Until recently, scientists thought the surge in brain pruning and wiring happen only once, when children are young. However, there is another surge right before adolescence. There is wiring of synapses which allow the receiving and sending of information. This is a critical and a sensitive period for growth and development for learning a skill or learning addiction and crime. Neurofeedback is a mechanism which treats depression and anxiety by recognizing the functional pathways in the brain. A depressed brain is fertile ground for many brain-based disorders like Alzheimer.

Practicing perseverance and creativity are among the intrinsic values to be instilled in brain-based disorders. These values interact with music and constructive emotions which are mutually influenced by the same area in the brain. Drugs are transported anywhere in the world, but the problem in Mexico is that it is a major producer and distributor of illegal drugs; it is a poor, overpopulated, and over-polluted nation which does not enforce the laws, and which seems to have difficulties when it comes to morals and integrity, ethics, values and discipline. There seem to be often a "Puente", fiesta, and a 2-hr lunch break which is quite striking for foreigners from North America who work around the clock. As part of the daily routine: cars are passing through red lights, ignoring traffic signs and rarely yield to pedestrians. The police rarely get involved in such "minor" legalities.

On the other side of the border, the US practices the bill of rights and the constitution in a well-organized and executive system which adheres to strict rules and regulations, striving for equality, freedom and a capital private market. However, the same values, if practiced irresponsibly, can cultivate a drug cartel such as in Mexico. Can the US battle Mexico's mentality or can it blend with this unique culture? Does it have what is needed to change it?

International Effect of Drug Trafficking

Palestinians

There is an analogy of the Mexican problem to the Palestinian and Israeli situation. There will be no peace in the Middle East as there will be no resolution to the drug problem in Mexico and the US. The Palestinians live in deprivation; in a ghetto; in occupied territories, with minimal living conditions, such as poor water and hygiene. They do not have the infrastructure for transportation, education, health, and agriculture. On the other side of the borders, Israel is built on high technology. Israel's construction is largely made by Palestinians.

In Israel, Hezbollah (a Sihai-Lebanese movement and terrorist organization) is founded on assassination. Hamas is another terrorist organization operating from the West bank, Gaza, and the occupied territories. Its fundamental strategy is suicide bombs and it is committed to Israel's destruction. These organizations are sponsored by Syria and Iran. It is clear that both organizations are disinterested in negotiation until there is an agreement to their terms and conditions which leaves Israel with a small piece of land. These terrorist organizations deny Jewish history and the existence of a Jewish state because millions of descended Arabs who fled Israel during the independence war have not been allowed citizenship.

In a documentary that aired on Fattah's Palestinian TV network, the narrator said "our (Arab) roots are deeper than their (Israel's) history", and therefore this should be an Arab state and not a Jewish state. Hamas exerts control on its people by confiscating donated humanitarian goods, forcing the Arabs in Gaza to pay for them. The Palestinian authority Hamas official Ahumad Bahr has updated the number 72 to 2.5 million virgins waiting martyrs. Muslim preachers have used the expression 72 virgins to encourage Arab youth to die in anti-Israeli terrorist attacks and suicide bombings.

With such determination, there will be no lasting solution in the Middle East. The majority of Palestinians and radical Arabs have no interest in two states living side by side. Unrealistic demands and expectations make this process impossible. Hamas wants a Palestinian state with East Jerusalem the capital. They want the Golan Heights and the territories Israel captured. They want Israel to allow Arab refugees who fled the country to return and also release all terrorists from prison. They want Israel completely out of Gaza, out of the west bank and the occupied territories. Once the Israeli Defense Forces leave, they organize mass destruction, and execute more terrorist attacks. If Israel refuses, they turn to their children to deliver their demands in the form of suicide bombings.

Children become their victims as they are unable to plan ahead and weigh the consequences. Children are impulsive to act. They rely on the amygdala, on the medial and temporal lobe to process emotions. They do not rely like most adults on the frontal cortex which governs reasoning and processes thoughts, because the prefrontal cortex is the last area of the brain to develop. The prefrontal cortex is responsible for organizing plans and ideas, forming strategies and controlling impulses. It is not fully developed until an individual's late twenties.

Disparities and inequalities bring hatred and envy. An article in Time Magazine showed pictures of Israelis enjoying themselves in cafés and lying on sunny beaches.[8] Economic gaps, resulting in envy and jealousy, mean a discrepancy between Jews' and Arabs' perception of discrimination and slavery.

Israeli construction is largely made by Palestinians producing these jobs. When the Arabs freeze the Jewish Settlements and decrease any further construction they hurt themselves. Being without a job means more poverty. The damage is mutual and causes intensified confrontation and tension between the two nations.

The United States

The US is under threat because it supplies Israel arms for it to protect itself and also provides monetary assistance. This leads to funding and support of the continuation of attacks and nuclear attack plans in Iran. This also leads to Al-Qaeda in Africa, promising Nigerian Muslims training, weapons, and money. The US exhausts resources to fight terrorism and drugs coming to the US. More tax money is used on security rather than education. The US tries to help Israel achieve peace,

---

[8]   *Time Magazine*, September, 2010.

but it does not seem that the Palestinians fully want it. The Middle East is not interested in peace. Likewise, Mexico really does not want to stop the trafficking, because some individuals do benefit from it. The Palestinians smuggle weapons much like trafficking in Mexico. Terrorism, drugs, criminals, and suicide bombers aim to harm the US and take control over our lives. Drugs and trafficking serve as a path for seeking power; an anti-social act, an outlet for frustration and an escape from reality.

Human trafficking cases are a concern for the two million worldwide who are affected. In the US, 15,000-18,000 individuals are trafficked annually while 10% of all prostitutes are minors controlled by traffickers. Reasons for trafficking are commercial sex and labor, housekeeping, agricultural and office work. Victims are put under conditions of slavery: overworked and having to endure hunger and heat. Many victims are young people from broken families. The sponsors show their "love" and "care" in the form of expensive gifts, promises and temptations. Traffickers prey on the victims' innocence, exploiting their weaknesses. Older men seek young girls and victims who cannot speak or answers questions for themselves. In this vulnerable environment when humans cannot speak, drugs can and this is fruitful ground for different types of addiction.

Who can lead, guide, and direct the Palestinians or the Mexicans if there is no one to trust? In Palestine, there is a long-lasting feeling of occupation and hostility. Hezbollah and Hamas keep planting seeds of rebellion and revenge. In Mexico, Mexican military and police distrust each other; they refuse to share intelligence and resist operating together. The mafia first pays the collaborators and then they kill them. Public and government officials who get involved often disappear suddenly.

Deception, bribery and corruption have become a second nature and a survival mechanism. Much like a pathological liar who uses lies to hide or cover the unpleasant truth, until it becomes part of his/her identity and s/he starts believing in his/her own lies; one lie creates another lie. Lying occurs because of fear of the consequences rather than taking responsibility, accountability, and learning to respect the truth in a productive way.

The Brain and
Behavior of Drugs

T HERE ARE SEVERAL myths surrounding the brain; the brain is not static as it used to be thought, there are no left/right brain individuals unless half of the brain is removed. Humans do not only use 10% of their brain capacity (it depends on the inactive areas), there is no drastic gender difference which implicates that either one should be taught differently. Learning experiences help the brain grow; however, nothing from the lab can imitate reality considering the fact that most of the research about critical age learning has been based on animals.[9]

Like in animals, the brain has a reward system that when a human engages in activities that help promote reproduction or survival (such as sex, eating, or nurturing behavior) it releases dopamine, which gives pleasure. The reward system is overly activated by drugs to the point that drug taking becomes more important than anything else because of the pleasure and reward associated with it. Newborns start life by relying heavily on the reward system.

Four weeks after conception, a human embryo is producing more than 8,000 new nerves cells every second. This is about a half million neurons made every

---

[9]   Bernard, S. (2010, Dec. 1). Neuro myths: Separating fact and fiction in brain based learning. *Brain in the News*, pp. 2-3.

minute during the first months of life. During the second trimester, the brain makes about 250,000 neurons per minute. In this critical period of development, the brain is making close to 173 billion synaptic connections. In the third trimester and through the first year of life, the brain develops and refines all the structures and regions that later make up the adult brain. New synaptic connections evolve, learning new information (semantic memories) and new experiences (episodic memories).

Another major neuron growth takes place again at puberty; nerve cells correspond to the chemical, hormonal, and physical changes of the adolescent body. Adolescents have trouble anticipating the consequences of their behavior because they rely more on the emotional amygdala than the rational frontal lobes. Teens become extremely vulnerable to addiction and adolescent addictions become harder to break. Teens are very susceptible to dopamine rushes of drugs that come with taking risks.

Interplay of neurotransmitters: Dopamine, Serotonin and Nepi

Drugs affect neurotransmitters in the brain. These neurotransmitters include; dopamine, which is involved in reward-driven learning. Dopamine takes part in learning, emotions, and attention as well as movements. Excess is linked to schizophrenia while insufficiency leads to Parkinson. Serotonin functions in mood, hunger, and sleep. Norepinphrine controls alertness and arousal. An undersupply of norepinphrine will depress mood.

Laboratory studies in a variety of animal species suggest that central nervous system (CNS) stimulants facilitate both the release of norepinephrine (nepi) and dopamine from CNS neurons. In humans, chronic administrations of high doses of CNS stimulants (e.g. amphetamines, cocaine) frequently produce a well-defined toxic psychosis that is often difficult to distinguish from paranoid schizophrenia. This syndrome, presumably due to chronic stimulation of dopaminergic pathways in the brain, is characterized by suspiciousness, hallucinations, paranoia, delusions; distortions in body image, hyperactivity, mood swings and occasional violence.

Dopamine and nepi are produced from the amino acid tyrosine. Serotonin and dopamine are produced from tryptophan. Tyrosine increases levodopa levels, which then increase dopamine levels and then increase nepi levels. Boosting dopamine to the right hemisphere can be done with crystal meth and cocaine to relieve certain conditions, such as ADHD, but creates other problems along with addiction.

There is interplay in stabilizing emotions among these three major neurotransmitters: nepi, serotonin, and dopamine. Depression blocks serotonin, while in ADHD there is insufficient nepi and dopamine, which are also apparent in social learning and autism.

Those primary neurotransmitters (along with sensory ones) are sometimes blamed for the confusion and misdiagnosis of autism. Autism shares some similar symptoms with schizophrenia, as well as clinical depression, ADHD, and epilepsy. Features of schizophrenia are inappropriate emotional responses, hallucinations and/or delusions, which are a result of GABA deficits, which leads to excess dopamine. Epilepsy is identified as seizures and loss of consciousness, which is a result of excess GABA which leads to excess of dopamine and norepinephrine. Clinical depression is marked by debilitating sadness, which results in a deficit of norepinephrine and serotonin. ADHD is interchangeable with autism for the over-activity and inattention characteristics of the two illnesses. Tics and Obsessive Compulsive Disorders (OCD) are also associated with a hyperactive state; tic disorders and uncontrolled emotional tantrums are seen in individuals at addictive states.

Obsessive Compulsive Disorders

Eating disorders, and excessive exercise, sexual activity, gambling, shopping, and Internet use, are all driven by loss of control. Addiction is an attempt to escape or cover the problem; it is an exaggeration and/or pre-occupation; and it is anything which undermines balance and moderation. Workaholism and obsession with money are just as much damaging as other addictions, such as gambling, sex, and substance abuse. When something is wrong people hope it will go away on its own and that they will not need to cope with it. When it does not, they repeat/sustain the behavior, which becomes an addiction by itself and the problem becomes more problematic.

People have to disconnect from materialism and take more time for themselves (e.g. taking a vacation) and reduce the stress with adequate reflection and nurturing. However people, such as nuns, who disconnect from materialism and devote and dedicate their entire lives to worship, may also encounter compulsion as a result of emotional deficits. There are periods through life that emphasis is heavily placed on one aspect to accomplish certain objectives, such as schoolwork or one's career, which are legitimate when they are temporary; but, an imbalanced lifestyle will cause problems in the long-run. Chasing after money and equating one's self-worth based on earning is debilitating and destroying. Capitalism is one of our nation's causes for addiction. Money does not solve the problem, it creates the problem.

A change in one's lifestyle is always welcomed, but it may be threatening, terrifying and paralyzing. People who had the same job all their lives, for the wrong reasons, may compromise their health and happiness. They often say "when I retire I will start something I really enjoy". This means they do not live fully and lack the effort to make a change. They look for better opportunities or alternatives, and are prone to develop addiction.

With a routine lifestyle (same places and people) it is easy to become depressed, empty, and unfulfilled. When people put their dreams and desires on hold until retirement they may never accomplish and enjoy them. In late adulthood they are struck by the fact that it is too late and they really did not exhaust their potential. Those who say, "of course if I did not have to worry about money I would have engaged in activities which I enjoy" fail to recognize the erroneous misperception that work and/or school must be unpleasant and serve as means to its end.

Our society does not show sympathy and tolerance for those who do not work or are not in school. For most employers, only the outcomes count. Our society does not care if jobs are stressful and create health problems; sleep or eating disorders; or anxiety and substance abuse. People in these types of jobs/situations may look for an outlet in the form of addiction. Our society does not care and employers call it an individual's problem, not society's problem

Food Addiction and Eating Disorders

Eating disorders arise from the difficulty that a compulsive overeater has with self-regulation, self-soothing, and from the mood altering effects of food intake on the emotional centers of the brain. Any food (not just refined and simple sugar) can have this effect. Certain foods replace or numb emotions. In shoplifting or gambling there is a similar adrenal rush.

For many, sugar and caffeine destabilize moods and increases the likelihood of cravings. Cravings for alcohol and sugar are the starving brain's way of getting a quick fix of the fuel it needs. The most significant change in treatments to stabilize moods and cravings is taking amino acids. Taking amino acids is a treatment that reduces the affects of eating sugar and caffeine. With taking amino acids there is a dramatic reduction in anxiety and depression, reduction of cravings, better energy levels and sleeping. Eating breakfast and having a diet higher in protein and complex carbohydrates also helps with cravings. Multivitamins and minerals, such as vitamins B and C are most needed to balance blood sugar. Once the amino acid has done the repair, there is no need for it any longer.

Food ingestion, much like smoking and self-administration of drugs, is linked to the neurotransmitter dopamine. A dopamine deficiency may be the main factor in drug addiction. Weight gain and weight loss are associated with addictive behaviors. In the past, the herbal drug known as ephedrine was used to treat obesity. Some experts believe that the addictive behaviors are a subset of OCD, and those with OCD are at risk for developing depression and other anxiety disorders. They also notate that many women who suffer from anorexia and bulimia become compulsive exercisers.

Compulsive Exercise

Compulsive exercisers tend to participate in extreme forms of exercise and eat erratically; a condition which results in numerous health problems, including kidney failure and heart arrest. Those who exercise compulsively have a hard time seeing there is a problem because exercise is socially acceptable and highly rewarded. Compulsive exercisers hide behind their illness. They maintain this illusion of good health due to the positive outcomes of exercise, rather than the negative; happiness is related to endorphins–the natural mood enhancing endogenous opioids, which are released during exercise.

Compulsive sexual activity

Compulsive sexual activity has similar characteristics to compulsive exercise; the level of natural endorphins is reduced in such addicts and they attempt to increase the level by constant sexual involvement. The normal pursuit of pleasure escalates or turns into an addiction because there is a problem in the brain circuits. Dopamine is probably not the only cause; serotonin is believed to be involved in the impulsivity that goes along with excessive consumption. It may play a role in compulsive behaviors. Individuals who exhibit a non-drug addiction have different serotonin circuits involved in their activities of compulsion.

Compulsive Gambling

Casinos drive gamblers to spend money by constructing a stressful environment and giving people the urge to control their environment. Tolerance to compulsive engagement in the activity of gambling requires "higher doses" and a huge personal cost to sustain the activity. Pathological gambling closely resembles all other addictive behaviors.

Major depression is a strong risk factor for the development of pathological gambling and for later relapse. Comprehensive treatment is required for depression or other coexisting psychiatric problems such as antisocial, narcissistic and borderline personality disorders. Major depression is also the predominant cause for compulsive shopping.

Compulsive Shopping

With shopping, buying something gives the addict a momentary sensation of wholeness when they feel empty inside. Researchers have looked at the financial, emotional, and environmental costs associated with consumption. Humans attune to cues that predict something that is unconditionally rewarding. They have great difficulty resisting these cues which contribute to addiction and relapse.

Internet

It seems that online there is a spellchecker and a contact list which makes information processing very simplistic, losing our ability to analyze with any depth. Most of us are ordinary people, who work from 8 to 5, with very little vacation time, and many responsibilities. Even when we get time off we tend to fill it with errands, Internet, videos, TV and texting. Texting requires less energy than an oral conversation and inhibits developing communication, social skills, interpersonal relationships and information processing. Excess Internet use is associated with ADHD and impairs social and academic development.

Texting is a debilitating cognitive skill, because when an individual multi-tasks, the quality of each task and the depth at which an individual processes information is diminished. Texting, like other Internet activities (including online gaming) can be clinically addictive because it offers rewards that those who are addicted crave.

Similarly, television addiction postulates that compulsive viewers turn to the screen when they are unhappy and unable to change their mood; they often watch far more hours than they intend, and not because they are bored. They may try to cut back on their hours of viewing, but find that doing so is difficult or impossible. Constant watching, much like excess Internet use, impedes a healthy social and family life. Studies have shown that excessive TV watching is also associated with overeating/obesity and sleep disorders. This can lead to the use of drugs which are approved for sleep disorders, but are erroneously used by healthy people. Provigil for instance is taken by those who wish to stay alert when they are sleep-deprived. There are no guidelines available for the use of such drugs by healthy people.

Pornography

When discussing Internet obsession one cannot ignore pornography. Addiction to pornography (including Internet pornography), sexual addiction, and other related compulsive and addictive behaviors, are related to depression, loneliness, and social isolation. Child pornography, in particular, may be an addictive behavior of pedophilia. Many addicts were sexually abused as children and are compelled to reenact scenes that they took a part of as children. Generally, sex addicts may enjoy sex less than most people because of the driven and compulsive nature of pornography addiction. It can also greatly increase a person's risk of unwanted pregnancies and getting sexually transmitted diseases such as syphilis, herpes, and HIV.[10]

Types of Addictions

Triggers and circumstances leading to substance abuse are: being repeatedly out of control; being subjected to and the target of stigma and prejudice; experiencing a life-endangering situation; damaged interpersonal relationships; losing financial, legal, or work status; medical complications; impaired well-being; and lack of resources.

Other mechanisms which interact with alcohol and drug abuse are an individual's value system and personality, expectations regarding the effect of alcohol or drugs, and genetic predisposition. These are often reflected in a family history, background, peers, the context in which drinking occurs, the availability of the drugs, the level of enforcement and local and national statistics.

Developing substance abuse and alcoholism varies with age of onset, social and psychological setting, and presence of psychopathology. It usually begins gradually without the people suffering from it realizing that they have symptoms of early addiction. Once they find their drinking is going out of control, they feel guilty, bewildered, and frightened. They attempt to rationalize each episode to explain their behavior to themselves and others. Their failure to regain control gradually destroys their self-esteem and the hope that they are worthwhile individuals. The response to this is similar to the development of other diseases; those that attack the integrity of personality, the ability to think, use language, and control feelings.

ANTI-DEPRESSANTS
Alcohol, Heroin, Opium-Pain Medications and Barbiturates

Alcohol

The ancient Greeks and Romans drank alcohol for both recreation and medical purposes, but advocated moderation in use. In the 13th century, the use of alcohol became common throughout western European society with an increase in the popularity of the distillation of alcohol. Babies born to women who engaged in moderate to severe alcohol use began to show symptoms of fetal alcohol syndrome. This condition, in its most serious form, caused physical deformities and mental retardation in the newborn.

---

[10]   Thakkar, V. G., Collins, C, & Levitt, P. (2006). *Addiction*. New York: Chelsea House.

Drinking during pregnancy can lead to a range of physical learning and behavioral effects in the developing brain, the most serious of which is a collection of symptoms known as fetal alcohol syndrome (FAS). The Wernicke-Korsakoff Syndrome is a result of alcohol damage to the brain. Up to 80 percent of alcoholics have a deficiency in thiamine and more of these people will go to develop serious brain disorders such as Werincke-Korsakoff. Approximately 80 to 90 percent of alcoholics with Wernicke's encephalopathy also develop Korsakoff's psychosis–a chronic and debilitating syndrome characterized by persistent learning and memory problems. People may not be aware that prolonged liver dysfunction, such as liver cirrhosis resulting from excessive alcohol consumption, can harm the brain which leads to a serious, potentially-fatal brain disorder known as hepatic encephalopathy. The two toxic substances of ammonia and manganese have a role in the development of hepatic encephalopathy. Damaged liver cells allow excess amounts of these harmful byproducts to enter the brain, thus harming brain cells.

In the 1960s, researchers found that new neurons are generated in adulthood. High doses of alcohol lead to disruptions in the growth of new brain cells. Fortunately, most alcoholics with cognitive impairments show at least some improvement in brain structure and functioning within a year of abstinence. Individuals with long histories of alcohol abuse have significant impairments in cognitive function due to brain shrinkage rather than brain atrophy. Deficits in learning and memory of neurologically intact alcoholics include impairment of visual perceptual functions, abstract reasoning and problem solving. It affects both men and women, and can persist for many years after cessation of drinking.

Alcohol works in two ways to slow down the brain's activity. It works by enhancing the function of the neurotransmitter gamma-aminobutyric acid (GABA), which is the main inhibitory neurotransmitter in the brain. Alcohol reduces the effect of glutamate (the primary neurotransmitter). After 1 to 3 drinks over an hour period the drinker feels decreased anxiety and stress, lower inhibition, pleasure/mild euphoria, and increased sociability. After 3 to 6 drinks the drinker feels dizziness, loss of coordination, poor memory, difficulty standing or staying awake, nausea and vomiting, and slurred speech. After 6 to 12 drinks the drinker feels hypothermia or hyperthermia, unresponsiveness with no movement, and shallow breathing which can lead to death.

Socialization, per se, does not reduce alcohol consumption, but under certain circumstances, isolation does. Experiencing drug-like effects is the primary motivation for continued alcohol consumption and alleviation of anxiety and depression. Social drinkers and chronic alcoholics experience anxiety and depression. It may produce either brief episodes of euphoria or a temporary amelioration of the negative affects associated with chronic intoxication. Alcohol intoxication appears to facilitate aggressive behavior; aggression is associated with plasma testosterone secretion. It is enhanced under increased interpersonal stress and/or losing status within one's social group. Plasma testosterone levels are suppressed in chronic drinkers during recovery following withdrawal.

When incorporating alcohol pharmacotherapy, a physician will prescribe either Naltrexone or Buprenhine, while also conducting an exam to look at vitamin deficiencies or unexplained signs of trauma. The physician may also conduct regular tests on the liver before prescribing Bupernorphine. Bupernorphine has some side effects such as feelings of discomfort or sickness that come with taking the medicine. Buprenorphine is an opioid with semi-synthetic components therapeutically used in the management of addiction and dependence to opioids including heroin, morphine and narcotic painkillers. It has a unique drug mechanism: unlike other opiates, it binds more powerfully to brain receptors thereby making it very difficult for other opiates to produce chemical reactions once Buprenorphine is taken. This drug prevents the withdrawal symptoms when a person stops using opioids like morphine and heroin by producing effects similar to these drugs.

A physician often prescribes oral Naltrexone if the patient is on Buprenorphine. Naltrexone is used to help narcotic addicts who have stopped taking narcotics to stay drug-free. It is also used to help alcoholics stay alcohol-free. Taking Naltrexone is an option when Buprenorphine treatment is discontinued. Unlike Buprenorphine, it does so without taking cravings away.

According to Eric Gunderson,[11] patients who maintain Buprenorphine on a stable dose may develop physical dependence, including withdrawal effects with abrupt cessation, but no compulsive and uncontrolled problematic use. Buprenorphine alone may not cure, but coupled with standards of care and psycho-social treatment it can produce long–term, sustained remission to alleviate the lifelong struggle for many individuals.

Among the drugs that are potentially available for treatment of alcoholism, lithium has two major advantages. The first major advantage is that physicians agree on the plasma levels required to produce therapeutic effects, and there are readily available methods for monitoring these levels in compliance with the treatment. Those who have medical problems (hypertension, heart disease, liver disease, etc) may need to take specific medications to avoid exacerbating their medical conditions. The fact that early signs of irritability and hostility are powerful predictors of later drinking and suicide in alcoholics offers an additional indication of the potential value of lithium. However, it has a narrow safety range and the potential side effects are many. As a mood stabilizer lithium can help control irritability, hostility, and feelings of suicide.

The symptoms of depression in alcoholics can be due to multiple causes, and therefore some interventions may be useful, but not others. Drug treatment

---

[11]   Gunderson, E. W. (2011, December). Buprenorphine induction: A major barrier for physician adoption of office-based opioid dependence treatment. *Journal of Addiction Medicine*, 5(4), 304-305.

produces a clear reduction in symptoms only in those alcoholics with high levels of anxiety or elevated Back Depression Inventory scores. Apomorphine has been used in the treatment of alcoholism for many years, not only to induce vomiting in aversive conditioning, but also to reduce tension and craving.

Naltrexone as part of alcohol treatment may not be suitable for patients with acute hepatitis or liver failure. Absolute contraindications for Naltrexone use are patients with acute hepatitis, liver failure, chronic opioid dependence or current opioid use, and active opioid withdrawal. Relative contraindications are for hepatic dysfunction, anticipated need for an opioid to treat an identified medical problem, pregnancy, breast feeding, severe obesity, and abuse during adolescence.

Injecting Naltrexone is considered when medication adherence is a significant concern in treating alcohol dependence. Opioid agonist treatment is the first line treatment for chronic opioid dependence that meets the DSM. Oral naltrexone and acamprosate are prescribed for patients with alcohol dependence. Successful treatment depends on self-help group support. The patient's improvement in health is related to non-drinking leisure and substitute recreational activities.

Heroin

Heroin is a precursor to morphine; it is converted to morphine inside the body. Although, the human body has its own opioid compounds, known as endorphins, many people do not produce sufficient amounts to combat their pain. The objective pain level (frequency, intensity, and duration) range varies in severity and the subjective perception of the pain varies in individuals. To enhance the natural opioids individuals can access, common artificial opiates are used in medicine such as morphine, codeine, hydrocodone, and oxycodone.

Injection of heroin causes the most powerful signal to the subconscious which signifies profound desperation. Addicts may experience slow mental functioning and extreme fatigue. Heroin addicts suffer from pneumonia, tuberculosis, and liver and kidney disease; HIV, hepatitis C, and other blood-borne diseases. Opiate withdrawal is one of the worst experiences, and is one of the reasons why opiate addiction is hard to break. Most of the heroin addicts want to get off the drug, but they are afraid to get off it because of the withdrawal effects—including the long sweat, the nausea, or the diarrhea. Heroin and other opiates have contributed to many premature deaths.

Addicts try to cure the withdrawal symptoms by using more of the drug. Acute administration of the drug provides brief euphoria, tension relief, enhanced sociability and elevated mood. There is also an increase in motor activity and a decrease in sleep. Opiate maintenance programs are controversial because they may give opiate addicts more opiate substances as a substitute, with the belief that they may help the craving and have fewer harmful consequences. However, the addictive potential is much less than that of heroin or other shorter-acting opiates.

Craving is described as an uncomfortable state of tension, accompanied by an urge to self-administer the drug. Increased craving most frequently occurs in the context of opiate withdrawal; however, in drug-free environments cravings may increase following exposure to stimuli that signal drug availability. These stimuli accompany the signs and symptoms of conditioned abstinence. The abstinent ex-drug user approaches an avoidance conflict (e.g. whether to use drugs or not in spite of the temptation). Chronic heroin use is accompanied by psychopathology, similar to what is observed in meth users.

Opioids

Opium addiction is based on strong cravings and loss of control. Craving occurs when the mind develops an overwhelming desire for the drug, and loss of control occurs when it becomes harder to say no to the use of the drug. Use is compulsive and continues even though the drug causes harm. There are some medical problems which are prevalent and more severe in people addicted to opiates than in the general population.

Methadone

The regulatory and weak antipsychotic effects of methadone may be particularly beneficial to opiate stimulant users. On the other hand, methadone and sedative hypnotic drugs produce synergic effects, which may make it difficult for opiate-sedative users to reduce their drug use and to concentrate on other aspects of their recovery.[12]

Methadone is often used in relapse. Methadone provides relief for those who do not respond to non-narcotic pain medicines. It has been used for decades to treat individuals who suffer from addiction and dependence on heroin and other opioid abuse such as alcohol, cocaine, marijuana, and tranquilizers. Antidepressants, cocaine and alcohol consumption during application of methadone are a particular concern due to the risk of death. Warning signs may have appeared only after the individual has left the clinic. The largest proportion of methadone use associated with death occurred during treatment; this occurred when the medical personnel overestimated the patient's degree of tolerance to opioids and the patient used other CNS depressant drugs in addition to the prescribed methadone. If a patient

---

[12]   Mirin, S. M. (1984). *Substance Abuse and Psychopathology*. Washington D.C.: American Psychiatric Press.

takes more doses of methadone faster than the body can metabolize it, serious toxicity or poisoning can result. Also, if a patient's methadone dose is increased too quickly respiration can be affected. To prevent respiratory depression, methadone should be administered cautiously to patients with medical conditions affecting their breathing. These include asthma, chronic obstructive pulmonary disease, heart disease (there must be cardiac screening for abnormal heart rhythm), severe obesity, sleep apnea syndrome, kyphoscoliosis, or a CNS disease. Patients who are new to methadone need to be told about the symptoms even if they do not purposely abuse medications or overdose. If symptoms or signs develop, patients should get medical attention immediately. Methadone can remain in the liver and other tissues, such as fat cells, from which it is slowly released back into the bloodstream. The slow release from these tissues may prolong the duration of methadone's action despite low levels in the patient's plasma. As with other opioids, methadone may impair mental and physical abilities required during driving and working, and therefore should be monitored.

When taken as prescribed, methadone is safe and effective. As all medicines, methadone may be more hazardous when used with alcohol, and other opioids or illicit drugs which suppress the central nervous system. The following substances— anti-depressant medicines, sleeping pills, antihistamines, tranquilizers, diuretics, antibiotics, heart or blood pressure medications, HIV medicines and MAO inhibitors—cannot be taken with methadone. Methadone maintenance is not an alternative that should be considered by anyone to whom other forms of treatment offer a reasonable chance of achieving abstinence.

Pain Medications

Addiction, psychopathology and pain are related, co-occurring, interdependent and compounding brain diseases. The symptoms of pain and common psychiatric conditions often overlap. Multiple specialists are consulted to determine the extent of an individual psychiatric or emotional deterioration resulting from long-term chronic pain. An interdisciplinary team specializing in patient care suggests that environment, nutrition, genetics and biochemistry contribute to the desire to self medicate. The environment constitutes work life, social interactions, family dynamics, peers, lifestyle and recreation.

Numerous studies have linked biochemical imbalances to nutrition, genetics, and self-medication. These imbalances included heavy metal, hormonal, and amino acid imbalances; methylation gene, hypoglycemia, histadelia, pyroluria, adrenal fatigue, thyroid disorders. Traditional treatments were based on personalized nutritional and diet plans such as amino acid therapy and supplementation aimed for food allergies. Other treatments that were used, which targeted healing the underlying causes of the symptoms driving the addiction (insomnia, depression, anxiety, mood swings, fatigue, racing mind, etc), were infrared sauna, Reiki, acupuncture, and gentle exercise. Addiction was determined by observation of repetitive, self-endangering and/or destructive behaviors. Tolerance and withdrawal were universal in prolonged opioid treatment. If sober living was impractical, methods of coping and adjustment also were taught.

Today a combination of cognitive-behavioral therapy, individual and family counseling, and nutritional bio-counseling are recommended. A comprehensive approach includes alternative modalities and techniques that address more than just the mental or physical component of chemical dependence. The goal is to bring together professional skills with holistic resources in order to create a comprehensive and integrated treatment for chronic pain.

Psychiatrists often ask how therapists could best serve patients suffering from chronic pain. Without medications, therapists encourage patients to abstain from all drugs and go to meetings when patients admit they are powerless over their pain. Therapists who suggest this to their patients are more successful than psychiatrists who take patients off one drug while prescribing another—the latter only prolonging their dependence. Pain specialists have traditionally had to deal with patients who desire to rotate off opioids. The dilemma today is still how to help these individuals achieve goals, without the use of medications, when pain itself is qualified as a psychiatric condition.

HALLUCINOGENS
Hallucinogens and Inhalants

Inhalants can be very toxic because most of them are not meant for human ingestion, but one of the greatest dangers is that the distortion of reality and hallucinations which come with the use of inhalants can cause users to be unpredictable. Hallucinogens, such as LSD, produce disturbances in the integration of sensory information, foster the development of perceptual distortions, and disrupt cognitive functioning.

The dangers of overdose from inhalants are brain damage (death of neurons, especially in the cerebellum), injuries to the face, mouth, throat, and lungs, burn injuries, irregular heartbeat, slowed breathing, lack of coordination, confusion, coma, and even death. There is little (if any) tolerance, dependence, or withdrawal associated with inhalants or hallucinogens.

Marijuana

At the time the Declaration of Independence was written (1776) cannabis and hemp were used in the paper on which the document was written. The first flags of the United States as well as 90% of American clothing were made out of cannabis; as well as the canvases of great paintings. Paper made from hemp was physically superior to that made from wood pulp. Hemp paper is still used today for bank notes and archives.

Since 1996, 11 states have passed medical marijuana laws, which made it legal for doctors to prescribe marijuana for their patients. However, marijuana has become the most commonly abused illegal drug. Marijuana, when it is not used for medical purposes, is illegal; it is the largest cash crop in the US, with earnings estimated at $32 billion per year. Mexico is the number one foreign supplier of marijuana to the US in addition to being a major supplier of heroin and methamphetamine. Chocolate products from the cacao tree stimulate some of the same receptors in the brain, but to a much smaller degree.

There is a panicked reaction in marijuana users' experiences, which cocaine and amphetamines occasionally trigger. That panicked reaction, or toxic psychosis, appears much like paranoid schizophrenia and may last longer among amphetamines users. Toxicity affects judgment and performance, and causes impairment of perception and motor skills, loss of memory and coordination. The more the individual has smoked prior to abstinence, the more profound the impairment.

Individuals who use medical marijuana because of cancer, severe chronic pain, muscle spasms due to multiple sclerosis and other painful conditions, are also prone to lung infection. Long-term use increases the risk of chronic cough, bronchitis, and emphysema. Users are more likely to catch sexual diseases and engage in risky behaviors because marijuana lowers inhibitions. Marijuana use increases the likelihood of patients engaging in activities that will lead to relapse.

Relapse is an inability to cope while the psychoactive drugs alter feelings and perceptions. The drugs make it possible for users to avoid dealing with unpleasant realities and to mask or dull pain and distress. Those who count on drugs to relieve pressure and pain find it difficult to deal with emotional and troubling situations. They slide into a pattern of avoidance, losing the ability to cope. Non-medical use of any drug may lead to compulsive, uncontrollable, and irrational use.

Marijuana use is associated with persistent detrimental cognitive effects. Marijuana inoculation has been shown to produce impairment of short-term memory, altered time-sense, increased reaction time, and a decrement in perceptual-motor coordination. Cognitive impairments resulting from smoking marijuana can last up to 28 days after the individual smoked the drug. Memory and learning problems caused by heavy marijuana smoking last for at least a week after usage has stopped; for the most part the problems disappear within a month. In terms of verbal memory, heavy marijuana users scored below the average on all measures of verbal memory, although they have no problems recognizing previously learned material. IQ scores on cognitive tests decrease as the number of joints smoked per week increases (and cognitive deficits persist after usage stops).

There are persistent reports of poor school performance in chronic cannabis users and trouble completing complex tasks that require sustained attention. Although, heavy users maintain a higher level of work output by smoking more, the behavioral placidity and feelings of detachment induced by cannabis use may function to modify hostile tendencies–particularly as they occur in certain interpersonal situations. Social drug use may limit the range of interpersonal contacts while solitary use may lead to isolation.[13]

STIMULANTS
Cocaine, Meth-Amphetamines, Nicotine and Ecstasy

All stimulants work through the neurotransmitters norepinephrine and dopamine. Stimulants allow both chemicals to exert a greater effect in the brain. Stimulants also have a significant effect on the cardiovascular system: they elevate heart rate, the blood pressure, and decrease appetite.[14] The stress the drugs have on the cardiovascular system put some individuals at risk of heart attacks or strokes and they can also experience seizures and even death.[15]

More volatile forms of stimulants are crack cocaine and crystal methamphetamines. Crystal methamphetamine is a growing problem since it is homegrown in the US. Cocaine used to be an ingredient in various tonics, including Coca Cola, throughout Western Europe and America. Other stimulants, like dextroamphetamine (Dexedrine, Adderaal) and methylphenidate (Ritalin) are used as treatments for narcolepsy and ADHD disorder. These stimulants are generally milder than cocaine or methamphetamine, although they can still have some of the same side effects.

Stimulants can lead to agitation and violent behavior. Addiction to stimulants has been plagued with violence and crime. Overdose is dangerous when a stimulant is mixed with a sedating drug, like heroin. A major adverse effect of stimulants is hyper sexuality, as a result of activation of the dopamine neurotransmitter system. This can lead to sexual assault and promiscuity. Craving for crack cocaine and other stimulants can be so intense that addicts become willing to do anything to achieve the next high.

---

13   Williams, J. S. *NIDA Notes*, Vol. 18(5), pp.1-4.
14   Health Services (2012, April 08) Princeton, NJ: Princeton University, p. 71.
15   Health Services (2012, April 08) Princeton, NJ: Princeton University, p. 72.

Cocaine

Although no clear evidence of physical dependence on cocaine has ever been demonstrated, cocaine users can develop profound psychological dependence with disastrous emotional, social, and financial consequences. Evidence has come, not only from behavioral observation, but also from biochemical tests showing lower levels of proteins which regulate synapses.

Consumers sleep less, eat less, and become addicted in a matter of months and sometimes weeks. Cocaine is considered a lifestyle drug–a drug which becomes a magical source of energy and inspiration. Cocaine reduces brain glutamate levels, and it has been found that treating animals with acetylcysteine reduces subsequent cocaine seeking. Acetylcysteine is a medication–a substance used to booster glutamate levels. Susceptibility to relapse occurs as part of administering levels of extra cellular glutamate associated with drug withdrawal. Glutamate is a neurotransmitter–a chemical that acts as a messenger between brain cells. Glutamate signals amplify addictive effects like in nicotine. Long term potentiation causes brain cells, which have been exposed to addictive drugs, to release dopamine more abundantly in response to subsequent exposures. Fluctuations in dopamine levels underlie the euphoria of initial drug use and contribute to other aspects of cocaine and other drug abuse or addiction.[16]

Once dopamine has attached to a nerve cell's receptor and caused a change in the cell, it is pumped back to the neuron that released it; however, cocaine blocks the pump. Those who use cocaine feel an extra sense of pleasure for a short time. Without the drug, the brain cannot send enough dopamine into the receptors to create a feeling of pleasure. The biochemical reaction cocaine causes in the brain (which affects dopamine production) affects joy, excitement, and fear. Paranoia and aggressive behavior are common. Overcoming the depression caused by stopping cocaine, while resisting the panic message from the brain, is a formidable challenge.

Many of negative effects on the heart can be also caused by cocaine's impact on the heart. Cocaine causes the body's blood vessels to become narrow, constricting the flow of blood. This forces the heart to work harder. When the heart works harder and beats faster, it may lose its natural rhythm. This is called fibrillation and is a dangerous condition because it stops the flow of blood through the body. Teens and young adults in their twenties are seen in emergency rooms because of the toxic effect of cocaine on their heart. Adequate doses of methadone may be required and enlisting family and peer support to cut down cocaine use. [17]

---

[16] Brain glutamate concentration affects cocaine seeking. *NIDA Notes*, Vol. 19, pp. 3.

[17] NIDA Notes, vol 20(5), pp. 8-10.

Methamphetamines

Meth users are obsessed with the effects of the drug once it becomes a part of their lifestyle. They become involved in pointless hours of nonsense activity which leads to delusions and exhaustion. Schizoid breaks, mental collapse, and physical deterioration are apparent.

Chronic use of methamphetamines can lead to auditory and visual hallucinations. Some people suffer from paranoia and delusions that bugs are crawling under their skin, and they may develop body sores from extreme scratching. Insomnia, malnutrition, hyperthermia (an excessive high body temperature), extreme rage, and precipitating violence are also common characteristics.

Chronic use of methamphetamines can cause inflammation of the lining of the heart. If users inject the drug, they may damage their blood vessels and cause skin abscesses. With the gay community, meth has enjoyed resurgence, becoming part of all-night encounters as a result of the drug's ability to allow long-term, desensitized erections and delayed orgasm.

Crystal meth is not the most addictive substance–crack cocaine and nicotine are more addictive. However, individuals who use crystal methamphetamines, which is typically more pure and thus a more powerful form of methamphetamine, are more at risk to developing psychotic symptoms that may persist after the drug has been used.

Men and women respond differently to treatment. Women who begin treatment for methamphetamine abuse report more psychosocial problems, and higher incidents of psychiatric symptoms such as serious suicidal thoughts and depression. They have difficulties understanding, concentrating and remembering, and show higher rates of prescribed psychiatric modifications. Although, women tend to begin treatment with more severe psychosocial problems than men, they seem to benefit from therapy more. Men report committing more crimes and have more involvement in the criminal justice system.[18] [19]

Methamphetamines users can achieve long-term abstinence with the help of community-based drug abuse treatment. It seems that young White and Latino unemployed individuals who are on public assistance, and/or those who have an arrest history benefit from a program which includes group therapy, mental health assistance for family, parenting and employment guidance.

Such programs help addicts learn healthy ways to deal with anger, improve communication, build social support and stay engaged in addiction prevention. Individuals reentering the community after incarceration require help with housing,

---

[18]   Whitten, L. Community-based treatment benefits methamphetamine abusers. *NIDA Notes*, Vol. 20(5), pp. 4-6.

[19]   Zickler, P. Brain activity patterns signal risk of relapse to methamphetamines. *NIDA Notes*, Vol. 20(5), pp. 1-3.

employment, finances, family relationships, and health issues, but only about 30% attend a treatment program regularly. Nine months after methamphetamines users attend the program they have reduced drug abuse, lower criminal activity, and fewer reports of depression. Many try to maintain or regain custody of their children by demonstrating improvement during treatment.

Meth treatment has moved out of specialized facilities, not only into community-based programs, but also into more routine health care. Young physicians are being trained to deliver therapy in a comprehensive treatment. Medications may help certain conditions: mostly behavioral, emotional, and physiological, but Cognitive-Behavioral-Therapy (CBT) and non-traditional therapy can compliment. Individuals with ADHD are often prescribed some type of methamphetamine for their conditions, despite the fact that meth is associated with cognitive deficits and poor academic performance. Ironically, the ability to ignore distractions can be impaired by consumption of methamphetamines. There appears to be a deficit in the ability to pay attention which undermines effective engagement in cognitive tasks. Scans of brain activity in methamphetamine users who relapse within 1 to 3 years after completing treatment indicate poor choices based on cognitive impairment.

Brain damage is observed by decreased blood flow in areas of the brain's parietal regions and in the frontal and basal ganglia regions. Activity patterns in those regions are also associated with relapse and are involved poor choices and impulsive destructive decisions. Increased blood flow in the parietal region indicates an increase in activity by glial cells. Glial cells shield and repair nerve cells that are damaged or exposed to toxins, such as drugs. These regions are involved in controlling response speed, attention span, as well as coordinating psychomotor speed and motor functions.

In a computer sequential reaction time experiment, participants pressed a key when they saw a number appear twice in a row (one-back target) vs. when a number repeated after one intervening number (two-back targets). On the one-back test, methamphetamine abusers average response time was 21.5 percent slower than non-users. On the two-back test the average response time was 18 percent slower than that of the non-users.

Methamphetamines may injure the brain's dopamine system, which is involved in working or immediate memory. A single-digit recognition test, that involves immediate memory, requires participants to press a key when they see a specific letter. There are consistently slower response times for methamphetamine abusers in tests that require working memory, immediate storage of information and mental concentration. In terms of motor function, brain damage that may not yet be noticeable in routine activities, but which is a more severe form of meth use, can produce symptoms associated with Parkinson's disease. This is a chronic neurological condition marked by physical slowness, tremors, unstable posture, and a peculiar gait.[20]

Amphetamines

Ecstasy is the most widely abused amphetamine among students and teenagers, because it is known for its mood-elevating, inhibition-lowering effect. The drug is associated with increased libido, euphoria, and inner peace. The damage to the brain's serotonin center, however, may be permanent, leading to severe depression. Methylene-dioxy-methanphetamine (ADMA), known as ecstasy, is a drug which destroys the nerve terminals of serotonergic brain cells. Serotonin is a chemical neurotransmitter that is critical for normal brain function. Disruption in serotonin levels are associated with psychological disorders that range from anxiety to depression and bipolar disorder.

Serotonin also plays a role in memory, cognition, anxiety, impulse control, sleep, and sexual desire. For children, the damage is even more dangerous because their brain is still forming. The drug causes lack of coordination, restlessness, confusion and poor concentration. About 6% of youth have tried ecstasy by 12th grade; the numbers are higher in college, and about 14 million Americans are current and former users.[21] Patients come to the emergency room agitated and not making much sense after they collapsed and were found by police or security. When agitated, they experience muscle breakdown because of the constant movement, which can sometimes cause kidney damage. Too little sodium in the blood could trigger seizures, confusion and arrhythmia. There is not enough known about the drug's long-term consequences and there is too little research. Some individuals are more vulnerable to long-term damage than others but it is difficult to predict who. Amphetamines, such as ADMA/ecstasy, are often taken with alcohol or other drugs.

ADMA has been used in talk therapy because it helped patients relax and open up. It helped them achieve insight, face deeply depressed thoughts, and analyze their feelings or memories. For similar reasons, ADMA has become very popular among high school and college students at parties. The number of teens/adolescents who have experimented with amphetamines has been on the rise, despite the fact there was no advantage to taking such drugs for those who had no symptomology.

Ephedrine has a chemical structure resembling that of amphetamines and produces similar effects. Cases of ephedrine abuse and dependence and the unregulated sale of patent medicines led to widespread opiate addiction. In the

---

[20] Zickler, P. Network therapy expands treatment capabilities of small practice providers. *NIDA notes: Research findings.* Vol. 18, No. 2, pp. 5-7.

[21] *Salt Lake City Tribune,* April 3, 2011, pp. 1, 6.

early 1900s the federal government instituted control over the sale and use of opiates (the Shanghai Opium Commission and the Hague Treaty) to curb the use and distribution of opium and coca. Such enforcement came from the Drug Enforcement Administration and the Narcotics division of the treasury department of the Internal Revenue Bureau. Those who inject the drug had an increased risk of contracting an immunodeficiency virus as well as hepatitis B and C. In addition, they developed pneumonia, tuberculosis, disease of the kidneys and the liver.

Tobacco and Nicotine

According to the Health World Organization, 5 million die every year from smoking, with 40% being children (500,000) who die from second-hand or passive smoking. In 2011, 1 billion people smoked tobacco as a result of emotional and mental events. Causes for death, besides complications of addiction, were physical: asthma, heart disease, cancer, and ammonia poisoning. One out of every six deaths in the US was a result of health complications related to smoking. The percentage of smokers age 17 or under who said they regret starting smoking was about 70%, and the percentage of youth smokers who continued smoking and died early from a smoking-related disease is about 30%. The percentage of smokers who started smoking in their teens is about 80-90%.

Adults who may start smoking in adolescence may have had a problem with low self esteem and were susceptible to peer pressure. They may have had problems with depression or anxiety disorders. Denial is deep even when addicts acknowledge that they have a problem and seek help to overcome uncomfortable emotions.

Acetaldehyde (a component in tobacco smoke) contributes to adolescents' tobacco addiction. Nicotine activates areas of the brain that are involved in producing feelings of pleasure and rewards. This partially explains why it is so hard for people to stop smoking. Nicotine is as addictive as heroin or cocaine. An individual is at risk for withdrawal symptoms when his/her body is dependent upon nicotine; the individual has adapted physiologically to the substance and now needs it to function. Chronic users report severe withdrawal symptoms, which make it very difficult for them to quit abusing the drug.

Nicotine cravings usually last for 3 to 5 days before another craving begins. Smoking harms the body because carbon monoxide binds to hemoglobin in red blood cells preventing it from carrying a full load of oxygen. Carcinogens, the cancer causing agents in tobacco smoke, damage the genes that control cell growth, causing cells to grow abnormally or reproduce too rapidly. Oxidative stress is believed to be behind the aging process, wrinkles in skin, and the development of cancer and cardiovascular disease.

The long term effects of nicotine for smokers who have used it for many years also include hardening of the arteries and atherosclerosis of the body, including the heart. Smokers have a much higher risk of strokes, heart attacks, emphysema, lung cancer, bladder cancer, and mouth and throat cancer. When nicotine is taken in combination with a different stimulating drug, such as cocaine, the effect of the two drugs together can cause severe vasoconstriction of the arteries around the heart and can potentially cause a heart attack. Sudden infant death syndrome can also result from second-hand inhalation and a mother who smokes. These infants did not choose to smoke. They became victims of their environment. Children of cigarette smokers and other family members of smokers are at risk for developing respiratory disease such as bronchitis, serious ear infections, and frequent colds due to their exposure to secondhand smoke.

Education is a preventive treatment factor among those who smoke, and more education usually means a decreased likelihood to smoke. Those with less than a high school diploma and those with high needs for dopamine are more likely to smoke. Cigarette smoking is common among former alcoholic and drug addicts. If they are smoking after they detoxify, they are more likely to relapse. Nicotine is a dopamine agonist and therefore seems to ameliorate some of the side effects of these drugs. Older antipsychotic medications are powerful dopamine agonists and cause many side effects. Treatment for a smoking addiction generally works when quitting with a friend or a significant other.

Clove Cigarettes, Bidis, and Additive-Free Cigarettes

Clove cigarettes, bidis, and additive-free cigarettes deliver at least as much nicotine as conventional cigarettes. Smokers who choose these types of cigarettes are as likely to become addicted to nicotine as are other smokers. They expose themselves to the increased risk of cancers, respiratory disease, and heart disease associated with smoking. The Smoking Machine Analysis reveals that clove products deliver more nicotine, tar, and CO than conventional cigarettes. Researchers attribute the clove cigarette's higher delivery of toxins to the lower porosity of its paper wrapper and its lack of filter ventilation holes, which are found on most ordinary cigarettes that dilute the smoke inhaled with each puff. After smoking clove, smokers had a comparable increase in the plasma nicotine levels, exhaled CO levels, heart rates, and systolic blood pressure as in conventional cigarette smoking. In fact, smokers took longer and more frequent puffs of the clove cigarettes than of their own cigarette brands. The analysis showed that two minutes after smoking, plasma nicotine levels increased the most for those who had smoked the additive-free brands.

Additive-free cigarettes are made with whole-leaf tobacco and contain no chemical additives, preservatives, or reconstituted tobacco. Many adolescents and adults believe that additive-free cigarettes are less harmful or less addictive than ordinary cigarettes, although scientific evidence contradicts that belief. Like clove-cigarettes, the additive-free cigarettes and bidis deliver more nicotine than do conventional cigarettes and, like the thicker clove cigarette wrappers, the bidis nonporous wrappers limit air dilution. Consequently, smokers increase their smoking as dependence increases, exposing themselves to greater smoking related health risks.[22]

Understanding Stress and Anxiety

The behaviors of drugs are governed by the emotional center of the brain; the limbic system and the amygdala. Hans Selye (General Adaptation Syndrome) hypothesized that when an individual experiences an intense fear and is incapable of regulating stress s/he is prone to illness. Those who cannot resolve the emotional turbulences may seek help in the form of substances and behaviors such as smoking. From here the "short-cut" to brain addiction does not take long.[23]

All new born babies start with 3 million brain cells that, through certain behaviors such as "college binge" drinking, are gradually destroyed. Once a brain cell is lost, it will not revive. Children from poor families have significantly higher levels of cortisol in their bloodstream. Children whose mother's show symptoms of depression display high levels of the stress hormone. A depressed brain is a fertile ground for Alzheimer's; the disease attacks faster with depressed patients as shown after autopsy. Depressed brains are riddled with brain plaque, sticky buildup around brain cells, and tangled protein fibers. One theory stipulates that when chemicals in the brain are not at a certain level and neurotransmitters are not balanced it can cause illness and some mental disorders. The theory advocates that medications relieve the symptoms by helping the brain chemicals stay at the correct level.

Anxiety becomes a concern when fears and worries make it hard to perform everyday tasks. No one knows for sure why some people get anxiety attacks while others do not. The emotional toll interferes with the capacity to capture the experience in words. It calls for psychotherapy interventions in the form of cognitive behavioral therapy. Prolonged exposure therapy; stress inoculation training; a cognitive processing therapy; acceptance and commitment therapy; a dialectical behavioral therapy; eye movement desensitization; reprocessing; motivational interviewing; and group therapy are all good alternatives for medications and work well in curing some of the symptoms.

---

[22]   Farrer, S. Alternative cigarettes may deliver more nicotine then conventional cigarettes. *NIDA notes*. Vol 18, No 2, pp. 8-9.

[23]   Hans, S. (1978). *The stress of life*. New York: McGraw-Hill.

Addiction-focused psychosocial interventions demonstrate that treatment is more effective than no treatment, considering prior treatment experience and preference. Possible psychosocial interventions include; a community reinforcement approach; contingency management and motivational incentives; motivational enhancement therapy; and the 12-step facilitation.

Writing about worries and stressful events helps with working memory. It is an effective way to communicate emotions through creativity and expression of emotional challenges. It opens the mind to the person's own beliefs and self-values. Addicts are taught to be mindful and not discount their feelings. Music is known to be a powerful stress reliever. While high volumes may evoke physiological stress response, low calm melodies give peace of mind. Addictive drugs and stress trigger similar change in brain cells, animal studies have found.[24]

Stress is a reaction to an unpleasant negative stimulus; addictive drugs, on the other hand, have a pleasurable effect. Relapse is reverting to a learned behavior. It is the effect of stress, like that of drugs, which plays a role in relapse. Long term potention (LTP) is one of the brain's key mechanisms for registering experiences and using it to shape future responses, as in learning and remembering. When an experience or other stimulus induces LTP in a brain cell, the cell responds more strongly to similar exposures in the future. LTP is part of the reason addicted and stressful/anxious individuals get excited the next time they are overdosing.

After months or even years of abstinence, former users may experience powerful cravings. Susceptibility to relapse, like the onset of addiction, is in part a consequence of changes to nerve cells in the brain. Most major drugs of abuse can induce LTP in dopamine-releasing cells in certain areas of the brain. Dopamine's roles include alerting the mind that something important is happening or about to happen, and triggering feelings of pleasure. Exposure to an addictive drug (amphetamines, morphine, nicotine, or alcohol) cause such pleasure, but drugs such as fluxetine and carbemazepine, which treat depression and seizures respectively, do not have such an affect.

Memory

People of all ages are sensitive to stress which narrows their attention. Cortisol, a hormone released during stress, is related to learning difficulties and poor performance on memory tests. Attention deficits can be reversed by removing stressors or teaching how to manage stress. An excess of cortisol from stress has been linked to heart disease, stroke, obesity and drug addiction. Stress hormones prime the body for the fight or flight response: increase heart rate, constriction of blood vessels, and a surge of adrenaline for energy. In approximately 25% of people,

---

24   NIDA Notes. Vol 18, No. 5. pp. 1-3.

these hormones remain elevated after the stressful experience. These people are at risk for developing PTSD. The longer the adrenaline surge lasts, the more vivid the memories become. In order to relieve the stress, the traumatic event has to be located in time and place, and be distinguished from the here and now. However, hyper-arousal intensity (or numbing) and dissociation get in the way of separating current reality from past trauma.

The accuracy of memory is affected by several factors, one of which include schemas—cognitive structures or frameworks that influence how new information is encoded, stored, and retrieved. Many distortions in memory are the result of interpreting information through existing schemas that may introduce systematic biases into memory. According to the trace decade theory, learning produces a trace or engram which incurs addiction. This is a physiological change in the brain that could decay over time as the result of disuse. However, in many instances memories are retained for long periods without intervening use or practice; this is seen when apparently forgotten behaviors are suddenly apparent. According to this theory, addictive behaviors can never be cured, although, this is not fully supported by research. Individuals with PTSD may demonstrate forgotten behaviors while they re-live the trauma again.

Periods of short-term memory loss are observed in post-traumatic states as well as in alcoholic blackouts and in certain seizure disorders and hysterical states. Blackouts result in impaired consolidation of new information, rather than repression motivated by a desire to forget events that happened. Neuroradiology and neurophysiologic studies suggest that there are transient changes in the neuropathological states commonly observed in addiction.

Does the brain work differently in some fundamental way when a person is using drugs, is abstinent, or is going through withdrawal? It can be seen if there is a functional effect of an intervention by watching the brain perform the same tasks before and after treatment. Developmental psychology stresses what is called the distinctive human capacity to link the self to others as a key trait of evolution. Mirror neurons bring about a revolution in the way humans see the brain, and the way they see themselves, their relationship to each other, and their collective awareness. Mirror neurons bring self-awareness by being conscious of someone else's consciousness to a certain behavior. Humans may be fundamentally interconnected, but they are also distinct individuals.[25]

---

[25] New technology expands the scope of NIDA's intramural Brain imaging program. *NIDA Notes.* Vol 18, No. 2, pp. 14-15

Alzheimer's

Every time a human mind wants to figure out how long something is going to take the brain samples from those time interval memories and picks one. Occasionally the brain pulls an outlier from that bell curve and may make the wrong decision. Individuals with less working memory rely less on the prefrontal cortex to do demanding thinking and reasoning tasks. The brains of regularly stressed adults ages 60 to 70 show a smaller hippocampus—the part of the brain responsible for learning and memory.

Alzheimer's disease, which is usually noticed at later ages, comes from a lack of the memory saving enzyme acetylcholine. Those susceptible to Alzheimer's have internal clocks that are saving memories from those clocks much more slowly. One common treatment for Alzheimer's memory loss is to take supplements that boost acetylcholine in the brain. These supplements can sharpen memory without giving the effect of caffeine because they never touch the dopamine system. As in addiction, the dopamine system in the brain is one of the primary causes of memory loss. Coffee and other stimulants make remembering easier, while an antipsychotic drug like haloperidol slows down the internal clock and makes a minute seem much longer and far less memorable. Marijuana is one of those drugs that interact with both dopamine and the acetylcholine system speeding up the former and slowing down the latter.

Medications approved by the Food and Drug Administration for Alzheimer's may not slow the disease's progress. The use of technology has a profound impact on new diagnostic tests. However, greater knowledge and awareness of dementia's symptoms will make early diagnosis more possible. Various ginkgo extracts are recommended for cognitively impaired adults, but the effects of these ginkgo extracts do not seem to apply for healthy individuals.

Aggression

People who drink alcohol are most likely to be associated with serious violent assaults. Amphetamine-based psychedelic drugs and marijuana have also been implicated in aggression. The best predictor of episodic violent behavior is a history of violent behavior. Addicts have a certain responsibility for the damage they inflict because they voluntarily make themselves irrational by impairing their judgment.

It is brain shrinkage, rather than brain atrophy, which is probably a function provoking aggressive behavior. Some individuals are unable to put the brakes on their drug-taking behavior when faced with potentially disastrous outcomes. In a healthy adult brain, the compulsions that flow from the activities of the insula and related limbic regions are normally held in check by the prefrontal cortex, which gauges the long-term consequences of behaviors. Addicts have prefrontal impairments (based on evidence from behavioral tests), making them more impulsive and less concerned about the long-term consequences of their behaviors. Studies have shown a reduced blood flow to the anterior cingulated cortex and the orbitofrontal cortex which make up around 5 to 10 percent of a healthy brain.

Multiple head injuries are linked to aggression, because brain injuries (particularly those causing a loss of consciousness) lead to problems in attention, memory, planning and behavior. Children and adolescents who have memory difficulties tend to get into trouble and have much more violent lives. Older individuals who suffer a head injury are on average five years younger when they are first sent to prison than those who have not been injured.

Brain Injury

Genetic and developmental factors as well as brain injuries can lead to a weakened prefrontal system, which makes some individuals particularly prone to drug taking and addiction. Diseases of the central nervous system put these individuals at risk of poor cognitive and psychosocial outcomes. Moreover, brain injuries cause problems in balance, walking and/or talking which get worse when a person uses alcohol or other drugs. There is most likely a relationship between reversibility of brain dysfunction and cognitive recovery.

The immature brain is susceptible to injury with long lasting cognitive and behavioral consequences. Individuals with brain injury score in the low average range on tests of verbal ability, and intelligence which is determined through performance on Intelligent Quotient (IQ) tests. Individuals with brain injury show deficits in executive functioning, abstract reasoning and attention, and have difficulties with mathematical skills and fine motor skills.

In addition to these pre-existing deficits in learning memory and language, these individuals are at risk of having related emotional and behavioral disorders. Other behavioral and emotional disorders which are typical to individuals with brain injuries are depression and anxiety, dementia and personality disorders. These individuals are likely to have poor self-esteem, diminished positive affect, high levels of stress, internalized behaviors, few family interactions, restricted social competence and independent behavior.

Children and adolescents with brain injuries are less adaptive to new stimuli and environments while older individuals with brain injury are less likely to socialize. Children and adolescents struggling with health issues may experience an increase risk for depression, disruptive behavior, and anxiety. They may be at greater risk for suicide than the general population, and be treated with selective serotonin reuptake inhibitors. Mental illness and cognitive dysfunction makes them prone to developing addiction.

Learning Disabilities

Fetal alcohol syndrome in the US counts for 50,000–70,000 children who are born with learning disabilities. Mothers make a bad choice if they drink during pregnancy, even if they take natal multivitamins or other prenatal precautions. Drinking and second-hand smoking have a detrimental effect on the fetus and on growing children. Children of alcoholic mothers (75%) fail to form lateralization. A longitudinal study, which took place for 7 years, revealed that more than 50% of children born to smoking mothers had learning disabilities, and more than 40% of them had ADHD. This was a result of failure to complete lateralization of the brain.

Most children exhibit brain lateralization, which is a preference to use the right or left hand. The left brain hemisphere is in charge of language skills, such as reading, writing, arithmetic, and fine motor skills. The right hemisphere is in charge of the emotional content of language, spatial-temporal relationship and the perception of shapes and music.

Two-thirds of right handed and two-thirds of left handed people develop language skills in the left hemisphere. The left hemisphere reads and the right hemisphere interprets. The right hemisphere understands people, which is important in everyday life and communication. This process is dysfunctional in autism. Changes in the right hemisphere may show problems in perception of shapes and understanding cues, resulting in dyslexia and depression.

Individuals with dyslexia have a large Broca's area in the brain and a high susceptibility to stroke. The Broca's area, located in the interior posterior area and which processes speech and language comprehension in the brain, is involved in expressive speech production and becomes enlarged resulting in slower reading performance. There is interactivity in the posterior-temporal-parietal cortex which effects sound and word analysis; and in the temporal-occipital cortex which deals with fast word recognition and memory. The production of speech is overflowed and imbalanced; it is never internalized, nor understood. Those with dyslexia have to learn sequencing in their speech.

The rise and fall of IQ scores appear to be connected to changes in the area of the brain associated with speech, whereas shifts in non-verbal IQ are related to an area involved in motor control and hand movements. For those in language therapy, the brain has to be in a receiving phase–shifting from expressive speech to receiving speech. The sentences have to be short. Those with dyslexia have to learn to listen and not interrupt. If therapy exceeds the capacity of speech memory, it does not allow them sufficient time to process. Their brain clock is slower in order to receive the information. Rewriting and asking questions about the content helps in processing information (read, retain and replace). Learning different alphabets and different letter structures from other languages can also stimulate their brain and facilitates language acquisition. Through kinesthetics, a child can trace letters in the air or make letters with his/her body. A child can be taught to deduct rules with non-verbal categories such as card games by sorting geometrical shapes into categories. The classroom is a noisy distracting place which does not help those with poor reading performance.

According to Brain in the News,[26] the brains of children with dyslectic processing styles are developing in different ways. Reading is more difficult for this type of child which makes pre-school a critical period for learning these skills. Children with dyslexia also may have difficulties picking up relevant cues from their surroundings and/or identifying voices over the phone without seeing the speaker. Children need help with distorted perception. Numerous therapies can substitute parents' reliance solely on medications; the medications that are usually a part of treatments can be addictive if not taken as prescribed. Dyslexia and ADHD do not imply addiction but certain behaviors are associated with these conditions.

Animal research

Drug abuse and overdose have been treated with more medications, resulting in more money being channeled into inventing medications to treat addiction. Medications have been formed and tested using animals, but the question has been whether or not self-administration of medications and research animals were reliable models of addiction and relapse in humans.

Animal studies have yielded fundamental insights into why people abuse drugs and how drugs cause the compulsion and disordered thinking seen in addiction. Animals have been used without exposing humans to potential toxicity, risk of addiction, or invasive medical procedures. However, animal research does not count for factors such as: diet, health, drug history, genetic makeup, socioeconomic circumstances, understanding and attitudes. In animal research, rats, mice, monkeys, baboons, and some other species are exposed to addictive substances in controlled settings. Conclusions are generally made based on coded observation of behaviors.

When baboons were injected with GABA-B blocker, they exhibited symptoms that included tremors, vomiting, and increased aggression, along with milder behavioral changes, such as assuming abnormal postures and sitting with their eyes closed, which were coded by researchers. The observations included time spent in resting postures and the animals' difficulties with tasks requiring fine motor skills. The symptoms increased with higher doses of GABA-B blocker and dissipated after its effects wore off. A slight increase in dose would tip the sedative effects to a lethal level.

---

[26] *Brain in the News*, October 2011.

Animals developed withdrawal symptoms when drug administration stopped: tremors, loss of appetite, and agitation were exhibited by the animals. In one animal research study, the animals exhibited addictive behaviors–they took more and more of the substance, devoted high amounts of time and energy to getting it, and continued taking it despite adverse consequences. They relapsed in response to environmental or stressful triggers and renewed exposure. Relapse occurred due to stress and environmental cues associated with the drug experience and exposure to the drug. Those treated with medications showed fewer signs of withdrawal than untreated animals when the drug stopped.

Humans rarely live and function in a controlled setting, and animal experiments can never yield a complete picture of how the human brain works and integrates qualities such as speech and writing, logics, and symbolic reasoning. Moreover, only in humans do social factors such as laws, culture, religion, and economics modify the likelihood and consequences of drug abuse.[27] [28]

---

[27]   Animal experiments in addiction science. *NIDA notes*. Vol 20(5). pp. 11-18.

[28]   Animal research shows GHB acts on GABA receptors. *NIDA Notes*. Vol 20(5).

Addiction and the Person

Addiction and Personality

DESPITE EFFORTS TO identify an addiction-prone personality, addictive disorders have not been etiologically linked to specific antecedent psychopathology. Heterogeneous groups of organic conditions were linked with an increased risk of addiction and more severe consequences. From the early days of modern psychiatry it has been suggested that drug abusers are not simply normal individuals who happen to be exposed to drugs, but that their compulsive drug use is symptomatic of underlying psychopathology. Most studies focused on personality attributes and used self-report personality measures to assess psychopathology. Few studies have examined clinical syndromes or psychiatric diagnoses in addicts. Thus, there was a gap between clinical psychiatry and addiction treatment programs.

A longitudinal study of drug abuse patterns brought attention to psychiatric disorders. Children were on average 6 years old when the study began and were subsequently interviewed at approximately 5 year intervals. Alcohol and substance abuse during the early years were significantly related to later psychiatric disorders—even after age, sex, parents' education, family income and episodes of prior psychiatric symptoms were controlled.

Early marijuana and tobacco use were each strongly related to participants' development of major depression disorders in their late twenties. Early marijuana use showed substantial effects on alcohol dependence and substance abuse disorders. "Alcoholic" personality used to be attached to individuals with defense responses, guilt, anger, and anxiety, and who had persistent impulsive self-destructive thinking. This thinking blocked a sensitive reaction to the danger of loss of control by drinking. Deviant children who became adult alcoholics seemed to have poor school success related to a high rate of truancy and low IQ scores.

In individuals experiencing withdrawal from stimulants: depression, anxiety, guilt, and low self-esteem were common symptoms. It was unclear however whether these signs and symptoms were a consequence of drug withdrawal, the unmasking of an underlying primary affective disorder or an expectable response to the social, financial, and occupational sequence of chronic drug use.

Three areas of psychopathology have been identified as consequences of addictive disorders that persisted beyond the period of alcohol and drug consumption: cognitive impairment, depression, and personality change. Where changes in brain function are a secondary effect of alcohol, it could also be a result of psychosocial consequences.

Brain researchers advocate that depression is a brain disease, rather than a chemical imbalance. It was found that brain pacemakers made depressed people happy again, because they stimulated their brains. Depression constitutes a special case in consideration of the relationship between psychopathology and addictive disorders. There are two types of depression: primary depression, which exists in the absence of other significant psychopathology or physical disorders, and secondary depression, which occurs as a consequence of psychopathology, alcohol and drug abuse.

Antisocial personality and depressive illness have been associated with increased rates of heavy drinking. Individuals who are diagnosed with antisocial personality disorder have a 15.5 percent risk of developing a drug abuse problem. People released from prison are less likely to re-offend if they do not use drugs again. It is difficult to discern whether the antisocial behavior observed in many substance abusers is a manifestation of a pre-existing underlying antisocial personality disorder or a learned behavioral adaptation to a drug abuse lifestyle. Although data suggest that family factors play an important role in the development of drug psychopathology in drug abuse patients, it is possible that some of the symptomatology is also related to states of drug intoxication or withdrawal.

In men, environmental factors such as behavioral modeling may play an important role in the spread of the disorder to their same-sex relatives. Men with strong genetic loading for alcoholism tend to have fathers and brothers that develop family alcoholism. In women, the presence of depression or anxiety, without drug psychopathology, appears to be an important impetus for the initiation of alcohol use and subsequent abuse. The development of alcoholism in females is less influenced by environmental contingencies.

There appears to be an environmental component to the etiology in mental illness. In sociopaths, however, there is evidence of pathological levels of cortical and autonomic arousal, and other neurological abnormalities. These individuals experience dysphonic moods and show evidence of impulsive behavior rooted in sensation-seeking attitudes and drug abuse.

Female felons with antisocial personality have significantly higher rates of alcoholism than those without antisocial personality. Female narcotic addicts with antisocial personality have a higher rate of alcoholism than do female addicts who are not antisocial. The behavior of these addicts is not just due to the need to support a narcotic habit, since they continue to be impaired even when they are not using drugs. Addicts who have personality disorders may be unaware of the problem with their behaviors which reinforces blaming and projection as defense mechanisms to avoid introspection.

Alcoholism and substance abuse are more prevalent in families of opiate addicts and stimulant abusers than in the families of depressant abusers. Those who later develop alcoholism have a history of heavy opiate use and ratings of high neuroticism. Other personality findings–such as schizotypal features in opiate addicts, borderline personality disorder and dependent personality in other drugs and alcohol–are also associated with neuroticism. Narcissistic, dependent, histrionic, and compulsive personality disorders involve serious neurotic traits which lead to impaired interpersonal functioning, poor academic achievement and difficulties with jobs.

Borderline personalities due to childhood trauma are very sensitive to rejection and abandonment and often respond to emotional threat by projecting their negative feelings on others or splitting the world into all good or all bad. If there is a history of sexual or other childhood abuse, they may engage in repetitive self-mutilation such as cutting or burning themselves with cigarettes–acts which are carried out to reduce feelings of anxiety and detachment.[29]

Addiction and Mental Illness

For the past century, schizophrenia has underlined a majority of mental illness. It has been defined as a psychosis and too little progress has been made for many people challenged by this disorder. In the brain, cells of the substantial nigra send signals to nerve cells that control movements using the neurotransmitter dopamine. Schizophrenia is affected by imbalance of dopamine, in the opposite way that Parkinson's disease is affected. In neurodegenerative diseases such as Alzheimer's and Parkinson's, there are two associating end-stages, loss of memory and other cognitive functions (in Alzheimer), and motor dysfunction (in Parkinson).

---

[29]   Williams, J. S. (n.d.) Early use of drugs may lead to later psychiatric disorders. *NIDA Notes*. Vol 18(5), pp. 1-2.

Good treatment rests on making correct diagnosis and identifying treatable target symptoms. An addict's drug of choice is a powerful indicator of his/her structural (ego-self) vulnerabilities and underlying psychopathology. Addicts' subjective feelings of distress and the relief they obtain from drugs remain among the most helpful guidelines when considering their treatment needs. Patients' problems with counter dependency, low self-esteem, self-care and self-governance are particularly amenable to the sustaining, nurturing, and organizing benefits of self-help groups. On the contrary, addicts with lifelong problems in regulating their rage and aggression will not benefit from a confronting approach.

Alcohol, tobacco and other drug addictions are related, but the fact that illnesses are comorbid does not necessarily imply a causal relationship even if one illness occurs first. Having an alcohol, drug addiction, or psychiatric disorder increases a person's risk of having other diagnoses. Usually those individuals have a lifetime history of at least one substance use disorder (e.g. alcoholics have a good chance to become nicotine dependent).

Nicotine, the addictive component of tobacco smoke, is as habituating as cocaine or heroin and it has a similar effect on chemical receptors in the brain. Smoking is prevalent among people with mental illness, which is often compounded by substance abuse disorders and alcoholism. Recent statistics show those with combined chronic mental illnesses die 25 years earlier than the rest of the population.

Addiction increases the risk that mental health problems will develop and the presence of other mental health problems increases the risk that addiction will develop. Excessive use of alcohol can lead to a condition known as alcoholic hallucinogens. Amphetamines can cause psychosis that is indistinguishable from schizophrenia. Preventing alcohol and other drug addiction halts comorbidity and increases opportunities for early, cost effective, and successful interventions in the presence of psychiatric disorders. Prevention works best where communities discourage use of alcohol and other drugs.

Schizophrenia is the disorganization of thinking and emotions, and therefore disordered thinking and inability to reason are characteristics of schizophrenia. Problems with the intellectual functions of attention, concentration, and memory accompany this disorder as it does in Alzheimer. Suicide is a concern for some people with schizophrenia. Some scientists think the illness begins before birth but does not show up until years later. This may further indicate that there are genetic mechanisms for these diseases. Individuals who are biologically predisposed to develop schizophrenia can do so by abusing drugs that bring about the onset of active symptoms. There are drugs that modify some of the symptoms, but it is still not quite clear what is going wrong in the brain.

Positive symptoms apply to people who are sometimes unable to tell what is real from what is imagined. Positive symptoms include: *hallucinations*–when a person sees, hears, smells or feels things that no one else does; *delusions*–when people on the radio and TV seem as if they are talking directly to him/her, when the person believes s/he is in danger and that others are trying to hurt him/her; *thought disorders*–the affected person has trouble organizing his/her thoughts and s/he makes up words that have no meaning; *movement disorders*–the affected person repeats motions over and over.

Negative symptoms include: dull voice, facial expression, trouble having fun, talking little to other people. Some symptoms resemble ADHD; having trouble planning, having trouble paying attention, and completing activities.

High creativity has not been linked to schizophrenia, as most people expect, but rather with mood disorders: notably bi-polar disorders or manic depression. Individuals with bi-polar disorder often attempt to alleviate their symptoms with alcohol or drugs. Judgment is impaired as the illness becomes active and the tendency to abuse substances increases.

One theory for schizophrenia is that people abuse drugs in an attempt to self-medicate the troubling symptoms stemming from the illness or from the side effects caused by medications used to treat the illness. However, some patients who attempt to self-medicate may possibly suffer from anxiety disorders, depression, or other psychiatric illness. Patients with schizophrenia and schizoaffective disorders who abuse substances or become addicted to them have high levels of impulsivity and sensation seeking. The prevalence of depression and substance abuse is significantly higher among the homeless. Patients who have manic episodes have a higher risk than patients with schizophrenia of having a substance abuse problem or alcohol addiction. High risk patients for addiction are also individuals with panic disorder, obsessive-compulsive disorder, ADHD and anti-social personality disorders.[30] [31]

Alcoholism and substance abuse both mimic and interact with all mental illness; to know substance abuse is to know psychiatry. For example, there is significant depressive symptomatology in opioid addicts, and trauma involved in alcoholism is a potential mechanism involved in personality change. The administration of low doses of alcohol improves a number of mood variables, but is lost with continued drinking. Suicide appears as a late complication of a long history of drinking or substance abuse.

A family history of depression without alcoholism does not seem to provide an increased risk of addiction for family members. However, children of non-alcoholic schizophrenic parents have an increased risk for developing alcohol problems in early childhood. Not all children with behavioral problems grow up to be alcoholics. These children sometimes have antisocial disorders, including persistent lying, stealing, vandalism, fire setting, and cruelty to animals. The symptoms were once thought to wane and disappear spontaneously in adolescence and early childhood.

---

[30]   Henderson, E. C. (2000). *Understanding Addiction*. University Press of Mississippi.
[31]   *Brain in the News*, December 2010.

This did not happen if their condition was associated with sociopathy, drug abuse, and/or addiction.

While childhood behavioral problems can be a risk factor for adult antisocial disorder and/or alcoholism, it is not clear why some children become alcoholics and antisocial adults while others do not develop either disorder. Childhood aggression and delinquency distinguish antisocial from non-antisocial alcoholics; alcoholic antisocial individuals report a higher level of those two than the non-alcoholic adults. Antisocial symptoms are predictors of job problems, vagrancy, violence and criminal activity. The abuse of depressants appears to be more closely tied to peer-influenced recreational use. It appears to be an attempt to self-treat some underlying psychiatric disorder (e.g. anxiety or panic disorder). Having an affective disorder does not increase the probability that the individual will have relatives with alcohol or drug addiction.

Discriminating factors are family history of alcoholism, childhood behavioral problems prior to age 12, hyperactivity and brain dysfunction. Behaviors which have been considered to characterize brain dysfunction/hyperactivity include: daydreaming, inattention, impulsivity and conduct problems. ADHD is often a second diagnosis; there may be prevalent delayed speech development, speech problems, poor coordination, and strabismus. Developing psychosocial and pharmacological approaches to treatment have addressed etiology focused more on social and cultural factors than on biological and genetic aspects.

In a patient with alcoholism and depressive symptoms, there are no reliable methods to distinguish which depressive and dysphoric symptoms are parts of a personality disorder, which stem from toxic effects of alcohol, and which may stem from some recurrent depressive diathesis. Many alcoholics who do not exhibit clear histories of major depression receive no specific treatment. Preventive treatment starts while the person's brain is still relatively normal.

Latino Adolescents

Beginning in early adolescence, Latinos and Native Americans lead the US in alcohol and illicit drug use. Among both Latino and non-Latino adolescents, psychiatric disorders have been found to be associated with the development of drug dependence. Research on the role of behavioral factors in the development of psychiatric disorders and the use of substances by Latino adolescents is sparse. The few studies that exist have found an association between substance abuse and the following factors: low religiosity, positive attitudes towards drug use, beliefs that drugs are not harmful, poor academic achievement and school failure. Participation in deviant behavior was also associated with substance dependence and addiction. Latinos were found to have disproportionably low income and low levels of educational attainment. Many Latino adolescents did not know that alcohol related car accidents were the number one cause of teenage death. They did not know that rates of substance abuse may be suppressed if they do not drop out from school.

Absence of family had a profound impact. On the other hand, "Familism" (a unique, defining trait of the Latino culture) was a protective factor against many of these negative factors. Positive self-esteem and problem-solving ability served as protective factors for the Latino adolescents. The higher levels of parental support (defined as praise, encouragement and physical affection) were considered shield factors against substance abuse.

Those who begin drinking alcohol during early adolescence are often introduced to alcohol by a family member. This is the social and cultural nature of most alcohol and drug consumption. Miscommunication with parents is a main factor, particularly in the face of the risk of drug use among Latino adolescents. Latino adolescents born in the US who have acculturated are more likely to exhibit problematic risk behaviors than foreign born and less acculturated Latinos. More acculturated Latino youth have higher rates of drug use than Latino immigrants. Cuban American adolescents have the greatest percentage substance use and significantly more illegal offenses than African American adolescents.

Parental substance abuse is associated with a higher risk of sexual abuse in childhood. Childhood sexual abuse appears to be common among Latina girls who abuse drugs. Many adolescents who are addicted and dependent on drugs admit lifetime abuse and trauma. The type of abuse, duration and frequency of the abuse, use of force, and the relationship of the abuser with the victims are associated with the number of drug abuse symptoms.

The impact of victimization is particularly harsh on those from poor, urban neighborhoods. Members of these communities have less access to psychological services. Drugs and alcohol is used as a way to distance themselves from the guilt and shame; facilitate social relationships; numb memories of abuse and compensate for the lack of personal power. The experiences of sexual abuse and the drug abuse bring them to therapy; however, more than half of Latinos using mental health services discontinue therapy after one session. One of the reasons is lack of bilingual and bicultural therapists. Social workers, developing and providing services to Latino clients, are not always aware of the cultural difference existing between the various major Latino groups. A trauma-focused intervention should pay particular attention to enhancement of self-esteem, the management of emotional pain, and empowerment of the adolescent.

Responses from Latino adolescents who took a drug knowledge questionnaire revealed some misperceptions which require further education. Some cultural misperceptions were 1) "smoking crack will not produce symptoms of cocaine use", 2) "regular cocaine use rarely causes addiction", and 3) "sharing drug needles does not increases the risk of contracting AIDS".[32] They were also not aware that increase in heroin use is closely associated with the increase in the number of injection drug-use related HIV cases. Given that the level of HIV among African Americans has been rising dramatically, in Latino adolescents the communication about dangerous activities has not been part of the norm.

Prevention messages are considered culturally grounded when participants can recognize the message as being about them and applies to their lived experience. Two conflicting needs preserve the culture of origin and yet become part of the new culture: adolescents' peer pressure against parents, and family respect. Culturally grounded and multicultural interventions may help adolescents deal with acculturation by encouraging successful integration into the new culture without losing their identity. A multicultural intervention can provide skills in drug refusal. Neglecting preventive measurements is likely to result in losing the protective effects of the culture of origin.

Poor school systems, economic disadvantage, and community violence do not address the environmental context in which these adolescents function and may neutralize the effect of positive influences. Ethnicity of the adolescent and alcoholism in parents are factors influencing the levels of stress in adolescence. Lifetime cumulative exposure to adversity and trauma predict risk of drug dependence and addiction. Successfully integrating culturally specific components in treatment must include staff members who speak the target population language and provide services in a culturally appropriate atmosphere.

Those who have immigrated to the US or who were born to immigrant parents feel greater peer pressure to engage in substance abuse and sexual activity. Mexican-American students report significantly more use of substances when offered by friends. They report using alcohol or drugs when they have sex. Alcohol is the most often mentioned drug of choice or first drug used, followed by marijuana and tobacco. Adolescents are unlikely to protect themselves if they are engaged in sexual experimentations. Adolescents who have been incarcerated as a result of delinquent behaviors are at a higher risk of engaging in sexually risky behaviors.

Contributing Factors to Addiction

Personality is an important factor in drug-using behavior, with respect to both drugs of choice and the propensity to become a chronic user. However, a culture which allows children to express their aggression and learned expectations related to drug use may be an important factor in how societies lost control over behavior. If an individual is told that the drug will make him/her aggressive, then the drug

---

[32]   Substance Abuse and Mental Health Services Administration (2012). Drug addiction: The emotional life (p. 126).

will probably do so. If s/he is told that it will make him/her sleepy, s/he will probably experience sleepiness. Epileptic individuals may be at a higher risk of alcohol abuse and/or dependence for the same reason.

Across socioeconomic, ethnic, and gender factors, family monitoring and rules have a stronger protective effect for males than females. Youths with low levels of family monitoring and rules are twice as likely to use drugs. Youth with low consistent family discipline are also twice as likely to use drugs. Youth with low family bonding are three times more likely to use drugs and youth with high family conflicts up to age 18 are over twice as likely to use drugs.

Family and peer factors affecting drug initiation are similar across gender and ethnic groups. Low levels of family bonding and high levels of peer antisocial activity are consistently associated with a higher prevalence of illicit drug initiation among young adults ages 12 to 21. Just having antisocial peers, especially after the age 15, increases the risk of drug use initiation (even after controlling for socio-demographic background, and prior alcohol, tobacco, or marijuana use).

Peer influence is found to be a strong predictor among female marijuana users. The quality of a relationship with a peer does not matter when it comes to substance use, but having a good female friend who uses marijuana influences the frequency of marijuana use. Boys in the 12th grade, in all ethnic groups, are more likely than girls to use marijuana, and there is an increased trend, especially with Native Americans.[33]

Friendship amongst females is critical to their wellbeing. After 50 years of research a study published by the University of California in Los Angeles indicated that there are chemical substances produced by the brain that help create and maintain friendship bonds among women. Women think, feel, perceive and analyze differently than men (In a Different Voice, Carol Gilligan). When women adapt to stress, the hormone oxytocin enhances relaxation, reduces fearfulness, and promotes care giving tendencies; Oxytocin enhances social contact and inhibits aggression. It was observed that women coped with substantial incidents by trusting their friends and relying on their advice, which in turn was proven to enhance existing emotional ties. Those who had true and loyal friends had reduced risk of major illness and recuperated faster. On the contrary, women without these established friendships did not show the same health results.

Some conditions increase a woman's risk for developing addiction. These conditions are: physical or sexual abuse, being a victim of past violence; having panic disorders, depression, and/or PTSD. The odds of a woman with PTSD to have substance abuse disorders are three times greater than a woman without PTSD. Women with drinking problems (59%) experience severe intimate partner violence in compared with women with no drinking problem (13%) which in

---

[33]   Relationships matter: Impact of parental, peer factors on teen, young adult substance abuse. *NIDA notes*, Vol 18, No. 2

return increases substance abuse. Both battered and chemically dependent mothers develop patterns of isolation, reporting few to no friends and very limited social and family networks. They experience shame and guilt for their situation and may be frightened that they will not survive. These women, who also may be mothers, are seen in society as causing or adding to the problems they will incur.

Rates of sexual and physical abuse reported by females in addiction treatment programs were as high as 75-90%, and 42% of domestic violence service recipients indicated they abuse alcohol or other drugs. In a recent survey, at least 25% of American women have been sexually assaulted and 18% of them were raped. Illicit drug use rates among women in violent relationships were 2 to 3 times higher than for those of in the general population.

In treating offenders in a community setting, those who relapsed to drug abuse had an extensive history of addiction, low rate of marriage, and substantial unemployment. The characteristics associated with high rates of relapse or recidivism are: being single, being without a steady job, and incarceration prior to treatment. Factors which were questionable in predicting whether any particular individual was going to become an addict were: IQ, parental socioeconomic class, competence, family function in childhood, emotional state, maternal supervision and mother-child relationships. Factors which were associated with future addiction were: school behavioral problems, lack of a cohesive family, lack of environmental support, less than a tenth grade education, being in jail and ethnicity (Irish for alcoholism). It became essential to emphasize family bonding and family monitoring, rules, and reduction of conflict at early stages.

Treatment helped offenders develop a sense of accountability for their behavior and as a result changed attitudes. The program was administered for three months during which participants learned about themselves. Each increase in the level of care was associated with a higher percentage of time spent drug free. A family history of alcoholism was a factor; if one of the biological parents was an alcoholic that individual had a four times increased risk of becoming an alcoholic even if s/he was adopted and grew up in another family where there was no alcoholism.

The problem with the statistics on the cases of addiction and their contributing factors is that data collection was primarily done by questionnaires and surveys. Respondents had to understand the meaning of each question, the administrator had to be the same, and the emotional state of those taking the survey had to be identical to eliminate mood swings. There was also the risk of social desirability in relying on survey results. In one survey, children reported a higher substance usage of phenoxydine, indicating an impossibly high drug use rate. The participants reported later that they were not entirely honest about the abuse.

Risk Factors for Alcohol vs. Protective Factors

Researchers have identified factors that put youth at risk for substance use and delinquent behaviors, and factors that protect children from behavioral problem. Among the risk factors are friends using substances and academic failure; among protective factors are bonding to family and community. There is a strong link between the behavior and these risk and protective factors, which are indicators of future problems and abuse as adults.

Among adults, risk factors are: easy retail and social access to alcohol, low enforcement of alcohol laws, low perceived risk of alcohol use, social norms accepting and/or encouraging drinking, promotion of alcohol use (advertising, movies, music, etc), and low or discount pricing on alcohol; disrupted family and relationships, alternation from pro-social peers, job and academic failure, negative work and school environment, low self-esteem and lack of social competence also apply to alcohol addiction.

Protective factors are: retailer education, compliance checks/sobriety checkpoint, parents' educating and monitoring, community programs, restrictions on advertising, family parenting skill training, social skill training, tutoring, changing work and school climate, communication, decision making and problem solving skill training.

Capital Factors for Addiction

Capital factors for any abuse or addiction are employment, health insurance, and personal status; these are also associated with the type of treatment chosen. Those who are least likely to use detoxification services are individuals with health insurance, recent employment, mental health service treatment and criminal justice involvement. Change in substance abuse behaviors is evident in those who use methadone maintenance and residential treatment. The factor most significantly associated with the use of methadone is health insurance. Employment is considered to be an enabling factor, because it can provide access to health insurance.

Age, race/ethnicity, homelessness, and parental status are predisposing factors for substance abuse. The predisposing factor "homelessness" is associated with three times likelihood of entering residential treatment for substance abuse (p. 167).[34] Among the inner city unemployed, substance abuse is often used as an antidote for boredom and frustration, as well as psychic pain. The use of drugs, in this way, has physical, psychological and social cost.

---

[34] DeLa Rosa, M., Holleran, L., & Straussner, S. L. A. (2005). *Substance-Abusing Latinos.* New York: Haworth Press.

Some individuals with addiction say these factors are negotiable, because politicians do not talk about drug abuse except as criminal behavior. Politicians and insurance companies like to see the individual as responsible for the problem, rather than finding responsibility with the public, the state, or the government. That way they can advocate that a lasting addiction is only a person's problem and not a societal problem.[35]

---

[35] Denizet-Lewis, B. (2009). *America Anonymous*. New York: Simon & Schuster.

Drug Abuse: Self-Medication or the Result of Experiences?

Understanding Depression

DEPRESSION AND ANXIETY are often associated with addiction. Substances may provide a temporary relief from stress and emotional pain: if the individual develops addiction as a result, this by itself may cause feelings of guilt and shame, and lead back to anxiety and depression. Traumatic experiences even in a past life or heritage can be a source for aberration/abnormality. An experience of having a distant father or a critical mother is sufficient to develop anxiety and depression. Once the person develops such an affective disorder, it is not uncommon to start using drugs in order to temporarily feel better; the drug modifies the balance of the neurotransmitters in the brain. Serotonin deficiency characterizes depression. With low serotonin a person becomes anxious, agitated, and restless. His/her vitality and ambition will be compromised with norepinepherine deficiency. Depression is manifested by dopamine and norepinephrine deficiencies and/or endorphin deficiency–the natural pain killer.

When endorphins are low, a person has difficulty feeling pleasure and may seek substances to produce that sensation. Deficiency of endorphins results in vulnerability to physical and emotional pain. When people hurt a person's feelings and s/he cannot get over it, this person becomes overly sensitive to emotional injury. This person is likely to become emotionally tired and will not be able to concentrate.

The fact that stimulants have an effect on ADHD disorders has made many individuals turned to meth for help with their depression. Most people focus better to some degree with stimulants, although as the dose of drug increases, concentration may actually become more difficult. ADHD is often interchangeable with depression. Depression is frequently an under-recognized factor that can impair performance in ADHD. ADHD can increase the risk of relapse because the drug is a "quick fix" that can make the depression disappear instantly. When the drug effects wear off, the brain has much less dopamine than before, and the depression becomes even worse than it was before using the drug. Drugs, such as crystal meth, release so much dopamine that they deplete the brain of its dopamine reserves. They prevent brain cells from producing more dopamine and are not able to replenish the depleted supply.

Addiction and Trauma

People are traumatized when they face a life event which they are helpless to affect the outcome of. Chronic tension, confusion, and learned helplessness may become typical responses to life as a result. Unresolved trauma damages the spirit and disables the ability to grow from life experiences. It creates splitting and numbness of self. Survivors alienate from the self and others and have unusual thinking and behavior, sometimes to the point of appearing psychotic. They tend to reenact or repeat self-defeating behaviors, exhibit sexual and somatic symptoms. Sometimes they will not talk about the trauma with others.

Silence is damaging to the body, mind and soul–"the body holds what the mind disowns"–resulting in physical discomfort. It serves as a cumulative stressor to the body, and the symptoms increase the probability of illness. As a result of the trauma the mind disables the creation of meaning, and often uses avoidance mechanisms.

Early trauma or an unresolved conflict situation leaves faulty circuitry in the mind. The mind relays traumatic experiences over and over, keeping constant stress signals running through the automatic nervous system. People with multiple addictions often have multiple traumas; they could be sexually abused, present in murderous behaviors, in wars or incest. The trauma could be someone else's experience. A woman, for example, lived with asthma since she was two years old. It was revealed that she had lost a younger sibling at that age; there was a connection between the asthma and the death of her sibling.

Addiction proliferates as the person dissociates—mentally separating him/herself from the body when the pain s/he feels is too great. The person feels detached of the body as long as the energy or pain of the trauma is there. A maladaptive coping strategy is to self-medicate; abuse of medications is a way to self medicate trauma.

However, when the medications wear off, the person starts feeling painful emotions connected with the trauma again and the pain is even more intense. S/he then wants to take more medications to detach from the pain and this starts another vicious cycle. The longer s/he stays addicted the longer s/he uses. The more intolerable the pain becomes the more difficult it is to get clean and get out of the cycle.

A withdrawal may be a threat to the self, which may draw the person to use again and abuse the drugs. The therapist has to work with the individuals on validation of their emotions, and their self-punishment for the occurrence of the trauma and the subsequent drugs use. Many of the painful images involve feeling alienated or abandoned, with these images often appearing in dreams.

Addiction numbs the painful reenactment of the core memories; however, the memories and the associated pain still remain. The person may already know the pain is not his/hers and may be trying to deal with it, but s/he may not be facing the problem. The trauma cannot be resolved if the person has a very cold and distant therapist or family members who have unrealistic needs and expectations. In transpersonal psychology a person is affected deeply by something that is not him/herself, but by those around them. Whether they are aware of it or not the person can pick up on a family member's thoughts and wishes, which are transmitted and prompt the person to obtain the drugs or drink alcohol. People do not realize that these are not their own thoughts/wishes, and think this is how they feel.

Self-healing with drugs may block the emotional and physical symptoms of the trauma by simply replacing one disorder with another. Some go to centers for alcohol treatment and come out addicted to Valium. Diazepam and other Valium-like drugs are the most dangerous to withdraw from and there is a high risk of seizure. These drugs, unlike others (aside from marijuana), are stored in fat cells, and are still in the body for a long time after the initial detoxification.

The individual that is reliving and dealing with trauma has to first ask what his/her life's destiny is; was the drug/medication necessary? When the father of an addict abandoned one particular patient, the patient did not talk about the abandonment; he had to regain back his lost confidence. Gaining emotional support is often an art in working on the negative experiences. Even when the addictive behavior stops the thoughts may still remain obsessive.

The dysfunctionality caused by the trauma has to replace the functional beliefs by saying, "I will no longer permit being abused" and "I am good enough". These individuals need to identify their need, not based on what others are doing, but based on integrity, strength and aloneness. Trauma separates the person from God, from one's self, and from others. Clearing the trauma and self-sabotaging negative beliefs enables the person to become more whole within, be more open, and work at a spiritual level. The use of substances may be an attempt of the person to connect with God: true prayer and meditation should come first.

Experiences in the intuitive body can be expressed in prayers and meditation. The intuitive body is what the Swiss psychologist C.G. Jung called the collective unconscious. This refers to the possibility of a later generation atoning to an injustice, without even knowing who the person involved was or what s/he did. The atonement of children for adults "to make it right" may be seen as self-sacrifice, or a compensation, which may end in drug abuse or suicide. [36]

Addiction and Post Traumatic Stress Disorder

Trauma leaves a sustainable, remarkable experience in victims' environment through five senses: hearing, vision, smell, taste and touch. Most areas affected by the trauma are the frontal cortex and the limbic system. The frontal cortex is responsible for abstract thinking, planning complex cognitive behaviors, personality expression, and decision making. The cingulated cortex is the basic circuit for communication, cooperation, empathy, emotional and attentional processing. It is activated when the individual is asked to be self-reflective.[37] It monitors personal, environment, and interpersonal information and allocates attention to whatever is most salient. The cingulated cortex is activated when people observe their allies experiencing physical pain, emotional suffering, and/or stress. The anterior cingulated cortex contains spindle-shaped neurons whose purpose is to connect and regulate divergent streams of information; the spindle cells are experience dependent. The anterior cingulated aids in development of self-control and the ability to engage in sustained attention to difficult problems. Those with larger anterior cingulated report more worry and fearfulness.

The limbic system is the emotional center of the brain. Once the victim begins to feel overwhelmed, s/he is in need of patience, empathy and understanding to recover. Traumatic experiences are stored in the limbic system, encoded into long-term memory through the hippocampus and the amygdale. The effect of the traumatic experience on the brain comes from shut down of the Broca's area (the speech production) and the Wernicke's area (language comprehension). Many individuals have no words to describe their experiences. There is a decrease in

---

[36]   Jung, C. G. (1981). *The Archetypes and the Collective Unconscious.* Collected Works of C. G. Jung, Vol. 9 Part 1. New Jersey: Princeton University Press.

[37]   Cozolino, L. (2006). *The Neuroscience of Human Relationships: Attachment and the Developing Social Brain.* New York: WW Norton & Company.

the hippocampal volume which causes memory disorders like fragmentation and dissociation symptoms. Hypersensitivity in the amygdala (processing and memory of emotional events) causes increased stress response, and hyper vigilance. Many individuals use defense mechanisms for self-protection (opposition, isolation, drugs, sex, and suppression).

The trauma is filed in the right hemisphere which is not only connected to language, but is also connected to emotional states, smells, sights, and touches. The trauma is remembered by repetition. The neurocortex looks for patterns and assigns meaning. The network of neurons is connected to the same concepts from filters. To change filters, new experiences and thoughts and feelings have to be experienced. All thoughts trigger a chemical; the chemical makes the individual feel, and then think based on those feelings. Thinking according to how the individual feels creates a state of being. The state of being gets interpreted as the individual identity; "after a long period of time s/he believes this cannot be change because to change our lives, situation or feelings would require changing who we are" (Joe Dispenza). Modifying social behavior is normally related to identity formation, and is based on modeling, patience, and relationship with the victim.[38]

It does not mean letting go to who they are, but rather letting go to who they are not: emphasizing the difference between what they do and who they are. According to Joe Dispenza, when the therapist provides love, support, and security, and when therapy repeats until new layers render, the experience no longer is threatening; the victim can forgive and let go of unneeded defense mechanisms.

John Biere's 6 steps of trauma processing stipulate exposure, activation, disparity, counter, extinction, and new feelings. New experiences can make positive new connections. Donald Meichenbaum proposes to help patients see what they did to make it to this point and what they have accomplished already despite of what happened.[39] Nietzsche stated that the purpose of life is "he who has a why for life can put with any how".[40] [41] Victor Frankl stated that life is also a higher power which may explain identity change–"suffering is the core of searching for meaning".

[38]   Dispenza, J. (2009). *The Science of Changing the Mind.* Health Communications, Incorporated.

[39]   Meichenbaum, D. (1995). *A Clinical Handbook/Practical Therapist Manual for Assessing and Treating Adults with Post-Traumatic Stress Disorder (PTSD).* Waterloo, Ontario, Canada: Institute Press: Donald Meichenbaum, University of Waterloo.

[40]   Nietzsche, F. (1954). *The Portable Nietzsche.* (Walter Kaufmann, Trans.) New York: Penguin.

[41]   Deleuze, G. (2006) [1983], *Nietzsche and Philosophy.* (Hugh Tomlinson, trans.). Athlone Press.

Helen Keller said "when the world is full of suffering, it is full also of the overcoming of it."[42] Her followers later stated that when love rules the world, there is no fear; every race and color reach out to each other, and turn an angry fist into a helping hand; there is no reason to fight, but willingness to listen and forgive; streets are safe place, kindness will appear on every stranger's face, and joy is in the heart of every man and woman.

Pets are often a source of joy and happiness. Military veterans when they are deployed find meaning in taking care of pets–which helps with the shutdown of their emotions, and communication. They live in a sustained "fight or flight" condition and feel under constant threat of death and injury. Some of the common symptoms are hypervilgilance, fatigue, nightmares, alcohol and binge drinking. They isolate themselves and once they return home they want to be alone. They may feel emotionally lost or feel they have lost valuable skills. In the battle field they may have lost their hearing, or have developed problems such as gastrointestinal, orthopedic, and/or sexual disorders. They try to adjust when their role changes, but their family may not be patient, open-minded and flexible.

Military prescription medications have more than quadrupled in the last decade. About five million prescriptions for pain medications, tranquilizers, muscle relaxants, stimulants and barbiturates were provided to troops in 2011. Alcohol and underage drinking developed another major problem in soldiers.[43] Drug abuse has become a habit in young soldiers and returning veterans. Veterans come home from war, holding memories which may make drugs appeal to them. They may abuse narcotics (heroine and morphine), benzodiazepines, marijuana, and stimulants such as cocaine and meth. When their body feels tired, they may try steroids to invigorate themselves. Returning veterans, ages 40-60, may have some pre-existing conditions and may benefit from medication.

Pharmacology can help improve sleep, but they may develop tolerance to the medications. The insomnia and stress may be perceived by the veteran as survival skills. Psychiatrists may recommend anti-adrenaline medications for the stress if they have no hypertension. A higher dose will be required to stop the intense memories, anxiety and depression. It puts insomnia into a question: whether the problem is physical or emotional.

Particular memories are uncomfortable and difficult to talk about. The memories provoke anger if the individual is not ready to talk or they are too fearful to share. Focusing on the cognitive aspect is very useful while integrating medications with psychosocial intervention. It is not always good to prescribe Celexa, Resperol, Trazadone, and SSRIs; it depends on pre-existing conditions because it may cause complications. Buporpin and malterone are anti-depressants which do not seem to be addictive, but may have some health risks for individuals with high blood

---

[42] Keller, H. (1996). *The Story of My Life*. Dover. Mineola, NY.
[43] *Deseret News*, September 21, 2012.

pressure, pulmonary hypertensions, and heart valve problems. They also suppress appetite, which contributes to weight loss. Other medications have an opposite effect and contribute to diabetes, strokes, osteoporosis, cancer, and dementia.

PTSD shares similar symptoms with Traumatic Brain Injury: seizures, alcohol and drugs disorders, concussions, and delirium. Therefore it is important to identify the problems related to each condition. Acute PTSD could involve panic behaviors and depression. Veterans with PTSD may not care what others think, because they have the mentality that their mission comes first; they "have to get the job done", and bring everyone else home safely. They have one identity (e.g. "I am a soldier"). When their military identity is broken or taken away from them, they sense emptiness and voidance.[44]

Reactions to trauma include: distressing thoughts and images; upsetting emotional or physical reactions to reminders of the traumatic experience. The trauma might feel to the individual like it is happening all over again. The individual is likely to avoid talking or thinking about it and go to great lengths to avoid reminders of the experience; avoidance causes feelings of detachment. The individual will always be on the "look out" for danger: s/he will be jumpy, irritable, angry, and have trouble sleeping. A common response of the individual to trauma is that talking about it will make it worse, and that it is better to forget it and move on: "I had a bad experience but I am just fine now". Traumatic experiences usually lead to experiencing medical and social disorders, and may be a crucial component in domestic violence, substance abuse, or mental illness. It is rare that an individual is "just fine".[45]

The trauma must be stopped and the recurrence must be prevented. Damage from the trauma must be repaired and healed. Any underlying or antecedent character weakness should be treated to prevent vulnerability to a recurrence of the trauma in the future. Shame and guilt can be intense and lead victims to suffer, isolate themselves or project of blame heavily onto others. Those who suffer from trauma use a variety of defenses: denial, magical thinking, minimization, grandiosity, and omnipotence. These defenses partly fail when the individual turns to drinking and substance abuse to blunt these feelings. Threats and damage to their self-esteem, stigma and social degradation, the devaluation of others, and the loss of status may prevent them from getting help. If a soldier tells a mental health worker, "I could not have a substance abuse problem, *I am* a marine. If you suspect this *you* must be poorly trained" or if a veteran says, "I am not an addict, just overworked", then there is very little that can be done until this individual admits and recognizes

44 Lieberman A. F., Van Horn P., & Ozer E. (2005). The impact of domestic violence on preschoolers: Predictive and mediating factors. *Development and Psychopathology*, 17(2), 385-96.

45 Cozolino, L. (2006). *The Neuroscience of Human Relationships*. New York: Norton and Company.

there is a problem. These individuals sustain terrible loss of integrity, self-esteem, crucial relationships, financial status, career, and health. Problem-solving capacity is blocked by cognitive impairment, demoralization, and lack of healthy coping mechanisms, but the greatest obstacle is the self-sabotage, the disruption and the reactive formation of denial.

Traumatic experiences may produce addiction. Addiction is a complication of the trauma effect of alcoholism and not a cause of it. In the pathological states of stress and trauma the following conditions may be met: dehumanization, recurrent terror episodes, death, loss of significant other, friends or family being killed, abrogation of causality and assaults on identity. Those with PTSD may experience a survivor syndrome; deny or avoid any recall of the experience, show isolation and apathy, express guilt and shame, and a need to justify their own survival. In addition to the survivor guilt and shame they cut all communication and exhibit symptoms of depression, somatization, and fear.

Abuse of Children and Trauma

Children can be affected as well as become victims of addiction. Repeated exposures to traumatic events affect children's brains and nervous systems. These events can influence academic performance, the engagement in high-risk behaviors, and difficulties in peer and family relationships. Traumatic stress increases health and mental health disorders, and increases the child's involvement with the welfare and juvenile justice systems. Once grown up they may have difficulty in establishing fulfilling relationships, holding steady jobs, and becoming productive members of society. Young children have the highest rate of abuse and neglect and are more likely to die because of related injuries. More than a third of criminal cases involve young children as maltreatment victims. Nearly two thirds of children in a Head Start program had either witnessed or been victimized by community violence.

Early trauma leaves the most damaging psychological marks, because there is loss of a secure base from a parent or caretaker. The impact of trauma on attachment is damaging to the child's expectations that parents can provide protection and comfort. The effects of maltreatment are elevated rates of aggression, over attribution of hostile intent; less empathy, lower social competence, lower IQ, poor language ability and school performance. Adverse childhood experiences determine the ten most common causes of death in the US. Adverse childhood experiences are the most basic cause health risk behaviors, morbidity, disability, mortality, and healthcare costs.

According to Lieberman and Van Horn,[46] children's response to domestic violence, witnessing violence and being the victims of violence shatter the confidence that their well-being matters and that adults will take care of them. The effects of exposure to violence are high levels of affect dysregulation, difficulty establishing relationships, reenacting the traumatic experience, sleeping disturbances, intense fear, uncontrolled crying, aggression and noncompliance. Sense of self and trust in others become permeated with fear, anger, mistrust, and hyper vigilance. These feelings conflict with the desire to have close relationships. Much of what causes time to be lost from school and work could be predetermined decades earlier by adverse experiences in childhood. Disregarding these behaviors as related only to a chronic disease or a self destructive behavior is detrimental.

The child's brain continues to grow and change long after the first new years of life and damage to the brain may cause childhood trauma. When the trauma repeats itself, high percentages of cells may die before becoming mature. Physical and sexual abuse during early childhood can short the circuit of normal brain development just as much as emotional abuse. Verbal abuse could be as damaging to psychological functioning as physical abuse. Verbal abuse includes teasing, ridicule, and criticism; yelling and swearing. Cruelty that is emotional rather than physical can come from peers as well as parents. Abnormalities in the corpus callosum, which is vital in visual processing and memory, indicate that emotional abuse from peers turns out to be as damaging to mental health as emotional abuse from parents. The neurons in the corpus callosum have less myelin; myelin speeds the communication between the cells. Neurocognitive difficulties are apparent with children who have been tormented by others. Studies showed fluctuations in levels of cortisol for such children. Boys who were occasionally bullied had higher levels of cortisol and girls who were bullied made less of the hormone due to chronically stress.

Bullying (even bullying that happens occasionally) weakens the functioning of the immune system of the person bullied and at high levels can damage and kill neurons in the hippocampus; this leads to memory loss and makes academic success difficult. Magnetic Resonance Imagery (MRI) studies revealed that teens who were bullied performed worse on tests of verbal memory than their peers and under-performed academically. Just a single session of being bullied is enough to have an impact on a child's brain.

Bullying can leave an indelible imprint on a teen's brain at a time when it is still growing and developing. This may cause reduced connectivity in the brain and sabotage the growth of new neurons. Bullied children are more likely to be depressed, anxious, and suicidal; are more likely to carry weapons, get in fights, and use drugs.

---

[46] Lieberman, A. F., & Van Horn, P. (2005).Toward evidence-based treatment. Journal of American Academy of Child Adolescence Psychiatry, 44(12).

Domestic Violence and Trauma

Diagnoses that accompany trauma due to domestic violence are usually depression, anxiety, ADHD, and conduct disorders. Risk taking behaviors are alcohol and drug abuse, suicide, eating disorders, delinquency, school truancy and suspension. The traumatic impact of domestic violence, until treatment is initiated, remains in the affective, behavioral, and cognitive domains. Trauma causes impairment in affect regulation, information processing, self-concept, behavioral control, interpersonal relationships, and biological processes. Affective symptoms are: sadness, anxiety, anger, emotional arousal, fear, and dysregulation. Behavioral symptoms are: avoidance, separation-anxiety, substance abuse, re-experiencing the trauma, oppositional behavior. Cognitive symptoms are: disordered ideas, harmful expectations of self, helplessness, worries, and concerns.

A child who experiences abuse is likely to be distressful; the distress may be overwhelming, and interferes with coping responses to other stresses, and promotes additional symptoms of maladjustment. A mother-child relationship is a mediating factor. Parents serve as models for relationships and social interaction as well as emotional anchors for children at a time of stress. A relationship-based treatment aims to enhance the parent's effectiveness as a protector: as a means of restoring the child's exposure towards healthy emotional, cognitive and social development. During diagnosis and the treatment process, the therapist looks at risk taking behaviors and levels of accountability, desire of the parent to change, openness, and parent's involvement in the child's life.

PRACTICE is one of the most recommended approaches for treatment; the acronyms stands for **P**sycho-education and parenting skills, **R**elaxation skills, **A**ffective-regulation skills, **C**ognitive coping skills, **T**rauma narrative and cognitive processing of the traumatic events, **I**n-vivo mastery of trauma reminders, **C**onjoint child-parent sessions, and **E**nhancing safety and future development trajectory.

The goal of affective regulation skills is to help the child and the parent learn to control their emotional reaction reminders. Cognitive coping skills focuses on changing cognitions about aggression and gaining control over the intrusive re-experience of the trauma. The goals of trauma narrative and cognitive processing of the traumatic event are: gradual exposure exercises, and verbal, written and symbolic recounting of the abusive events. The child learns to be able to discuss the events when s/he chooses in ways that do not produce overwhelming emotions.

The goal of in-vivo mastery of the trauma reminders is to encourage the gradual exposure to innocuous/harmless trauma reminders into a child's environment. The child learns to control his/her emotional reactions to things that are reminders of the trauma–starting with non-threatening examples of the reminders. The child-parent sessions deal with psycho-education, sharing the trauma narrative, anxiety management, and correction of cognitive distortions. The parent works to enhance communication and create opportunities for therapeutic discussion regarding the trauma. The goals of enhancing safety and future development are: training and education with respect to personal safety skills, healthy sexuality and interpersonal relationships; it encourages the utilization of skills learned in managing future stressors and/or trauma reminders.

PRACTICE is effective for children who shut themselves down, normally between the ages 3 to 5 in response to parental and social invalidation of their emotional needs. As they grow-up and pass from early childhood to late childhood and adolescence, they experience changes in their neurochemistry. Having a unique perspective is especially painful during this time when everyone is trying to fit in. Children at these transition may become easily overwhelmed and it may be surprising the lengths they are willing to go to avoid the pain.[47]

---

[47]   Marohn, S. (2003) *The Natural Medicine Guide to Addiction.* Charlottesville, Va. Hampton Roads.

Addiction and its Effects on Family, Children and Teens

Growing With Abuse: The Addicted Family

ANY ABUSE CAN cause damage to a child's sense of self and his/her ability to self-regulate painful emotional states. A child may view sexual activity as a coping strategy, and as s/he grows older s/he develops a sexual addiction. Women with addiction to alcohol or drugs have a higher incidence of sexual addiction than other women; this sexual addiction may be due to childhood abuse. Addicted women who are victims of childhood abuse are required to identify core beliefs and basic assumptions that underlie behavioral choices and allowing for conscious changes in the behavior. They have to identify and address the developmental problems that occurred in childhood as a result of abuse.

As a child grows up in a family with addiction, s/he might have difficulty experiencing intimacy with others. In a state of dependence, relationships feel less secure and anxiety increases. Those who grow up in families with addiction often unconsciously seek out a partner who has the same kind of problem, because that is what they are accustomed to. These individuals are usually women with borderline features and codependency. According to the Diagnostic Statistical Manual, borderline individuals show impulsive behavior, intense and unstable interpersonal relationships, unstable self-image, feelings of abandonment and an unstable sense of self. Co-dependent individuals become emotionally invested in relationships with individuals who are not functioning independently and are addicts. Borderline features and codependency are often found in the relational style of those who develop depression and anxiety. As the addicted individual suffers, the entire family suffers. Among these types of families, there might be marked increases in domestic violence, child abuse, depression, anxiety, and illness.

A burden is placed upon a child when parents come to the child with their emotional needs, which increases the child's anxiety and interferes with the child's psychological and mental development. In dysfunctional families the parent-child role is likely to be reversed, and children may feel responsible for the family function. These children are denied age-appropriate needs in the interest of the family's functioning and survival. The way a child responds to stress and the negative forces within the addicted family shapes his/her behavior and self-concept. Children raised in an addicted family exhibit low self esteem and depression; inability to identify emotions; poor conduct and academics; underachievement, and delinquency. Some respond to tension and conflict in attempt to control others.

Sometimes it is not the child but the spouse who gradually takes over the responsibilities that the addict is failing to assume, and becomes "the enabler". The enabler's behavior is motivated by love for the addict and for the family and wishes to compensate for the addict's mistakes. A burden is placed upon a child when parents come to the child with their emotional needs, which increases the child's anxiety and interferes with the child's psychological and mental development. In dysfunctional families the parent-child role is likely to be reversed, and children may feel responsible for the family function. These children are denied age-appropriate needs in the interest of the family's functioning and survival. The way a child responds to stress and the negative forces within the addicted family shapes his/her behavior and self-concept. Children raised in an addicted family exhibit low self esteem and depression; inability to identify emotions; poor conduct and academics; underachievement, and delinquency. Some respond to tension and conflict in attempt to control others. Sometimes it is not the child but the spouse who gradually takes over the responsibilities that the addict is failing to assume, and becomes "the enabler". The enabler's behavior is motivated by love for the addict and for the family and wishes to compensate for the addict's mistakes.

Addiction in the family is a relapsing disorder, which means that some periods of abstinence may be followed by a return of the active addiction. A permissive, non-restricted environment and psychological pain are both factors in relapse. Life in an addicted family is likely to be unpredictable and chaotic. Addicts may minimize what's happening, because it would be too painful to admit the truth.

The family also resists threats to change in the status quo. Parents blame the school system and resent therapy.

Feeling guilt or anger the family members may wish to keep the peace rather than discuss their true feelings. Denial of those feelings allows for disconnection between bad memories and the associated emotions. Impairment in emotional and interpersonal functioning is masked by an attempt by the family to appear normal to the outside. The family resists threat to change in the status quo. In addition, the addicted family has a tendency to assign and displace blame to others. Parents blame the school system and resent therapy. The "do not talk/ do not feel" attitude restricts what emotions can be felt; all emotions are passed through a filter. There may be an unspoken ban on the expression of strong negative emotions and on causing conflicts while dealing with the addict's behavior.

The Effects of Domestic Violence and Addiction on Children

Addiction and domestic violence share many common features, and pervasive social and health problems. They cut across all demographic categories, tend to become progressively worse over time, and are potentially life threatening. They are often intergenerational, and affect all members of the family; domestic violence typically involves denial by all parties, and results in isolation of the individuals and families, and involves additional problems (e.g., legal and financial).

It is not clear what comes first–the domestic violence or the addiction. Nor can one implicate that either one is the cause for the problems. When the family is in chaos and there is no communication within the family, due to a lack of listening and conversation skills, violence seems to be a convenient instrument to attract attention.

The effect of domestic violence on children includes increased odds that children will enter school without cognitive, social, emotional skills and other competencies. Those children who are placed in special education may drop out before graduation, and have difficulty with their grade retention. Common struggles of children from addicted violent families are: making and maintaining emotional relationships, the feeling of being different than others, and seeking approval and affirmation. When expectations for children of these families are too low and they are told that they are a failure, they tend to confirm their behaviors to their parents' low expectations in the absence of meaningful support.

The emotional and behavioral effects of violence on these children are: emotional liability, aggression, hostility, destructive behavior, inappropriate sexual behavior, and regressive behavior. Children living in domestic violence are not only subjected to unrealistic or unsafe expectations, but also at risk of homelessness, hunger (which leads to the use of food banks), poor health (which leads to a need for medical care), and admission to foster care by child welfare services.

Children living in domestic violence tend to report: truancy, running away from home, and substance abuse; along with eating problems, pornography addiction, sexual assaults and harassment. Addicted family members become preoccupied with drugs and alcohol, show increased tolerance and binging. They loss control, have blackouts; lose respect for themselves and other family members. They neglect themselves, and are likely to have problems at work. The family may experience psychosomatic illness and depression. Addicted family members may suffer memory problems, extreme indecisions, tremors and fears, and may try to escape the violence. The family becomes suspicious, "walks on eggshells", and may be socially withdrawn. Good parenting is virtually impossible in such environments. If the substance behavior could not be used or performed, the individual feels physical and psychological side effects.

Domestic Violence and Mental Health

Families which live in domestic violence compulsively protest the display of negative feelings and only positive feelings are okay. Numerous subjects are taboo and there are many secrets within the family. Everyone must conform to the strongest person's ideas and values. Punishment and shame prevail in an atmosphere of unclear and inconsistent rigid rules. The atmosphere is tense and consists of anger and anxiety. The entire family is tired and exhausted.

When growth is discouraged, the family demonstrates low self worth and coalitions exist across generations. Each child exhibits different feelings and behaviors based on their place within such families; *lost children* in the addicted family are hurt, angry, lonely, and inadequate, have poor self-image, disconnected and afraid. The *scapegoat child* is fearful, lonely, hurt, rejected, and jealous. The *mascot child* is fearful, insecure, confused, lonely, anxious, helpless, and tensed. The scapegoat and the mascot children are at a high risk of suicide.

Mental disorders are frequently present in these individuals at the time of suicide (estimates from 87% to 98%). Mood disorders, most of which are cases of depression, are present in 30%, substance abuse in 18%, schizophrenia in 14%, and personality disorders in 13% of the suicide cases. Numerous medications are substantial for these mental disorders, but these medications can also be a source of abuse. Seroquel is an anti-anxiety medication to treat mental illness. Other useful medications are Vistrail–used as antihistamine and for anxiety; Wellbutrin–an antidepressant which is easy to overdose on; lithium–a mood stabilizer; Haldol and Risperdall–long acting typical entophytic. Nicotine is an anti-seizure medication, but in the case of abuse, smoking cessation is required. Malingering is often exercised by female patients for insurance and social security purposes. They show no objective signs for illness, hallucinations or manic episodes.

Acute and chronic substance abuses are associated with an increased risk of suicide. Substance abuse is the second most common cause of suicide after mood disorders. Often destructive behaviors, such as cutting and self-mutilation, mask a stress response to abuse, sexual assault, or sexual identity confusion. Cutting may be a standard outcry for attention, though there may also be suicidal ideation.

Mental health providers and domestic violence experts should plan treatment collaboratively. Assessments of substance abuse in youth and children should include domestic violence screening. This ensures more client-centered approach, accountability, and comprehensive holistic approaches. Individuals with brain injuries, that are a result of domestic violence, may have hallucinations, visual problems and developmental disabilities. Family members who live in domestic violence appear to have poor cognitive abilities or mental deficits; discipline and behavioral problems; as well as high drop-out rates from work or school. Hostility and destruction against family members may cause them to take a dysfunctional role as the scapegoat. In addition to the presentation of anger and unrealistic expectations, there are issues of trust, resentment, frustration, and chronic fatigue. Their fear becomes their own debilitating thoughts related to going back to school, being unable to find a job, expanding their internal world, and fulfilling their emotional needs. The therapist or clinical administrator can make referrals to appropriate agencies to better coordinate care, child/legal protection, parenting and training.

Once the family completes the intervention program successfully they are considered "recovered". Recovered families are able to freely talk about negative feelings and are open to discussion. Family members feel they are accepted and members are responsible for their own actions. The rules are flexible, the atmosphere is relaxed, there is energy, joy, and all family members work together through stress. When the family is in recovery, growth is celebrated; the family gains back its good condition, self-worth and a strong personal coalition.

Domestic Violence and Substance Abuse

Every 15 seconds a woman is beaten in the US and those who live in violence, also practice violence and become violent. Women who suffer from domestic violence tend to drink and use substances. Substance abuse does not cause domestic violence and domestic violence does not cause substance abuse. There is only a relationship between the two. Family chaos and domestic violence are related to drug abuse, but family violence does not necessary stop when substance abuse stops. However, both affect family members and involve denial, social isolation, use of power and control. They may cause emotional numbness and chemical dependency.

There is no justification for substance abuse. Substance abusers use excuses possibly due to shame and guilt. Many who experience domestic violence use meth, heroine, and cocaine. They relapse and victimize themselves by saying, "I am powerless in all aspects of my life". Some of the misconceptions in these individuals are that they may die anyway and therefore the substance cannot hurt them much more. For instance, most smokers began their habit when they were in their early teens. If the substance behavior could not be used or performed, the individual felt physical and psychological side effects.

Drug therapy which is FDA approved is usually recommended along with family consultation and some other form of psychological treatment. Medications are recommended when appropriate. Medications work modestly, but psychotherapy also works moderately; behavioral modification works in about 8%. A combination of medications, psychotherapy, self-help and participation in a professional support group seem to be more effective. These treatments improve cognitive impairment and coping skills with proper exercise and nutrition. During treatment, family members should be asked about their daily routine, and should be in a contingency therapy which gives external rewards.

The treatment for substance abuse related to domestic violence has been controversial partially because brain disorders are involved. Clinicians have had to provide increased understanding, planning and screening. There is constantly new research looking at the brain to see how it functions: not only for substance abuse, but also to study stress response, the release of dopamine, and the glutamate systems. New drugs bring novel approaches, and a need for medication development, genetic testing, behavior and physical testing.

One eighth of men who commit acts of domestic violence also have substance abuse problems, according to a survey conducted in 2009. In the same survey, female victims reported that they started abusing drugs or alcohol following the start of their relationships to the offenders and because of their male partners' substance abuse. The men may have turned to battering their partners to forget, and the women may have begun to drink to relieve the pain. Engagement in domestic violence and substance abuse numbs emotions and guilt.

There is a false assumption that battered women are co-dependent and thus contribute to the continuation of the abuse; but, treatment is recommended not only for women who are primarily affected by domestic violence, but also by the batterers. Ninety-five percent of reported cases of domestic violence involve a male offender and a female victim. Male offenders who may be perceived as "tough" guys could be very soft inside and can enormously benefit from treatment by becoming educated about medications and community resources. Treatments that recognize and utilize that softness include playing with cooking materials such as rice to reduce stress, writing songs about their acts and singing it to the person's affected by those acts. Battered women must get sober before they can address their victimization and not become refugees of casinos, which facilitate drinking and gambling addiction.

The therapist should also be aware and seek information about the family of origin of the abuser to uncover childhood abuse. It is very likely that the abuser was abused by a significant other as a child. Victims would have PTSD like symptoms such as: numbness, disconnection, anger, irritability, sleep disturbances, fear, and guilt; feelings of worthlessness, social isolation, mistrust and alienation. Those with both, PTSD and substance abuse, have a more severe clinical profile than those with either disorder alone.

Domestic Violence and Substance Abuse in Children

Many youths and adolescents apparently turn to substance abuse because of serious underlying psychiatric disorders. Depression is usually the major illness in alcoholism. Sometimes the depression predates the alcohol abuse. At other times the depression may be triggered by alcohol abuse. Children adopted as older children are likely to exhibit addictive behaviors or mental illness in adolescence and adulthood.

Children are considered a high risk population, because they are either at a disadvantaged from a socioeconomic stand point or because of other factors associated with the family. High risk children live in environments that are considered high risk because of disruption or dysfunction. Families may be dysfunctional for various reasons such as physical and sexual abuse, and/or emotional illness of the parents. However, even functional parents may face serious problems in dealing with children who have special needs or other problems that lead to addiction. In both cases, the poorer the relationship with their parents, the more likely the child is to start a relationship with drugs.

The term high risk has been used in reference to children who: grow up in urban, crime ridden environments, under conditions of poverty; and with parents who were ill-equipped to nurture them. Children of overworked and exhausted parents, who have little unscheduled time, may be left unsupervised to experiment with drugs. Parental alcoholism and drug abuse are risk factors for children's alcohol and drug use. Permissive attitudes toward drug use are just as important (or more important) than the parents' actual drug use. Alcohol and drug abuse can exacerbate the problem in young families who generally have less money than those in middle age. These children have little hope of breaking out of a vicious cycle of school failure, delinquency, drug use, teenage pregnancy, and chronic unemployment. Children who are at risk for abuse and neglect are also at risk of dropping out of school, becoming unemployed and/or becoming premature adolescent parents.

A child's lack of contact with their parents, lax supervision, absence of parental demands, parental disinterest, or lack of affection for the child are detrimental and further the development of substance abuse disorders and addiction. Children with conduct disorders and those who are runaways are also at high risk for alcohol and drug abuse, regardless of socioeconomic background. Signs of conduct disorders can be predicted starting from 5 through 7 years of age. Among those signs are: acting out, impatience, impulsiveness, defiance and negativity. The later inability to become attached to others in a healthy adult relationship ("don't talk, don't feel, and don't trust") brings a sense of isolation and abandonment, and may even produce shame.

Girls complain about abdominal and back pain, and show symptoms of psychiatric disorders. Some become pregnant or begin using alcohol and drugs in an attempt to create significant attachment and gain affection. Boys report that they perceived drinking as a release from pressure, a celebration of independence, and a mature behavior. The main reasons reported are: relief, an alteration of conscious; and release from anger, inhibition, judgment, or worry. The earlier the drinking starts, the more likely that child will have sex at an early age, use narcotics, smoke, fail in school, be involved in legal proceedings, and develop alcoholism. Young boys, who seek out help for a drinking or drug problem, need the interpersonal communication skills that enable them to seek help for themselves and/or their families. The families of these children are socially isolated due to the shame; the families live in a state of disorganization, and are unable to conform to social expectations. They may well deny any problems and dismiss confrontation. The core problem is the family's sense of alienation and isolation and, above of all, inadequate social skills to bond and communicate effectively.

Atmosphere of extreme tension and argumentativeness in the family seems more upsetting to the child than the abuse per se. Therapists and mentors can develop or clarify family rules for children and implement them accordingly. Family factors are the strongest influence for delaying or diminishing the initiation of children's alcohol and drug use. Alcohol and drugs are the nature of fighting, mistreatment, neglect, and broken promises. Many parents who have busy and erratic lives do not examine their family life, and participation in family activities suffers. Also, when alcohol is perceived as more important to an addicted parent than the child, the parent gives-up the child to his/her peers and to the high risk environment.

Children use alcohol and drugs as a means of peer pressure, to be accepted to and identify with a peer group in order to feel like they fit in. For them, drinking is getting drunk. Strong family connections with the examples of role models can support in resisting the pressure, while bad role models are more likely to lead the way in beginning alcohol and drugs.

Children need to be taught that there are many ways to feel valuable and important, and that it is important to talk to trusted adults. There are caring adults who want to help these children feel valuable, important and secure. They can establish open responses to sustain and broaden discussions and expression of feelings without passing judgment or blame. Children of alcoholic parents can be high achievers, bright and over-responsible because of their stressful home environment. Adolescents today spend more time away from the family, and have more social and economic pressure placed upon them. Family activities narrow to watching TV and movies. The messages on the screen for beer, wine, and liquors become as big a factor as the increased availability to alcohol and other drugs in the family environment.

Many parents say that alcohol and drugs are a national problem and may be unaware of the problem in their own homes. The attitudes of parents towards alcohol and drugs may make it difficult for them to take positive actions to prevent use among their children. Permissive parents allow their children to smoke marijuana at home and believe that occasional use of drugs is not risky. Once they recognize they are losing their child and their child is getting into trouble, it may be too late to seek help and to start setting a goal and work towards that goal; it may be too late to share their problem with others and find assistance. Parents should be helped by healthcare professionals in order to reach out to their children, before the stress of the situation creates the need for the child to escape to alcohol and other drugs. Parents should be provided with information on specific drugs and their effects. The family may feel less informed than their child who gets drug information from their friends, and they may find it difficult to talk to their children about substance abuse, dependence and addiction.

Parents need to utilize statistical information to better understand the probability of alcohol and other drug use by their children. Some parents may think their children do not take certain drugs because they do not have the money to buy drugs. Parents may have little information about the harm of specific drugs. They should be alerted to the effect that certain transitions, caused by drugs or the onset of adolescence, may have on their children's behaviors and feelings, and be encouraged to talk with their children about these transitions. During transitions parents should stay involved with their children's activities and school programs; know their children and friends; and provide a role model for a healthy drug-free lifestyle. Parenting seminars, school and religious programs, and audiovisual materials are a valuable resource because they allow demonstration of roles and parenting techniques. Parents should be given the message that validates their important role in prevention of alcohol and drug use. It is important that they know as much or more about drugs as their children are likely to know, and that they recognize the signs and symptoms of alcohol and other drugs use.

There is a need to have resource packets to help families adjust and instruction for skill building to help parents communicate with each other and help their children develop social competence. Therapy in a group format is not a good option for parents' involvement because of its high turnover of members; as children grow parents may move out of an age-appropriate group. These are some other alternatives. Groups may also be inexperienced in organization management.

Children can easily overdose on drugs and die of a fatal overdose. Overdose of over the counter cold and flu medications have caused some teens to die within a few weeks. The inhalation of solvents, glues, and other cleaning agents can cause everything from brain shrinkage to bone marrow loss over the long term, and oxygen deprivation, heart arrhythmia, and memory loss in the short term. Methamphetamines are prescribed to some children, especially in schools, to treat their ADHD. Methamphetamine prescription is viewed by some psychiatrists as a form of child abuse because in many cases the drugs are misused, cause dependence, addiction, and health complications.

Children who present with first time seizures at the emergency room should be evaluated for amphetamines abuse. Droperidol and haloperidol may be prescribed; these drugs are both antipsychotic medications that treat hyperactivity or agitation and are used to terminate amphetamine-induced seizures. Other medications are used for hypertension, hypotension, hyperthermia, and metabolic electrolyte abnormalities.

Joseph Biederman, a psychiatrist at Harvard University, has found that bi-polar disorder and conduct disorder are much more predictive of alcohol abuse than is ADHD among adolescents. Sexual assaults occur more commonly when alcohol is involved. Overall, assaults and addictive behaviors that are related to alcohol, tobacco, and drugs abuse are commonly reported among low-income and less educated families.

Adolescent and Teen Culture

According to the 2011-2012 nationwide survey on substance abuse in adolescence there has been an increase or unchanged rate of abuse over the past decade of some prescription drugs, inhalants, and other substances in 8th, 10th and 12th graders. Overall, the use of heroin and hallucinogens by teens is on the rise. Survey data does not indicate long-term decline in the abuse of illicit drugs either including marijuana, among 8th graders; and only indicates a very modest decline among 10th and 12th graders.

In one of the surveys,[48] 21.4% of high school seniors admitted to smoking pot in the past 30 days. After marijuana they were most apt to use prescription and over-the-counter drugs. A participant in the survey testified that he tried marijuana in ninth grade. He said it was casual; he felt guilty and worried that he would be caught. Later, he also did spice and mushrooms, alcohol and tobacco; he learned to deceive his parents. Over time, his means of escape became bigger.

---

[48]   *Deseret News*, August 5, 2012.

The consequences were more demanding. His grades plummeted and he started skipping classes. Forty-one percent of 12th graders report having had a drink in the previous 30 days and by the time they reach college that number climbs to seventy-two percent. Approximately 200,000 adolescents visit emergency rooms each year because of drinking-related incidents and more than 1,700 college students die every year.[49]

Adolescents tend to drink differently than adults. About 90% of all teen alcohol consumption occurs in the form of binge drinking, which experts say peaks at age 19. For many teens, the point is to get drunk, as quickly and cheaply as possible, in part to reduce the social anxiety rife at that age. Adolescents show much more frontal cortical damage than adults. One high dose of alcohol causes significant loss of brain stem cells. When teens start drinking early, they are 40–60% more likely to become alcoholics, regardless of family history.

The brain's dopamine system peaks in adolescence. Differences lie in the immaturity of the rewards system in adolescents' brains, such that it is overly active especially in response to novelty. Their sense of themselves and how they are perceived by others is falling under the executive control or impulsive control. Those who have trouble controlling their impulses are most likely to experiment with drugs and overdose. Combining energy drinks, which can have far more caffeine than coffee or cola, with alcohol is particularly a problem. They are much more likely to be injured; much more likely to be taken advantage of by someone sexually; and much more likely to drive drunk.

Teens and adolescents also are highly vulnerable to the effects of overdosing on anabolic steroids. Dr. David Simonson, a counselor and relationship expert, suggested that teens and adolescents used alcohol and steroids to feel socially accepted, to "fit-in". Anabolic steroids can be very dangerous to teens and weaken the immune system, leading to liver damage or cancer. They can permanently stop bones from growing in teenagers, impair learning and memory, and cause mood changes escalating from depression, irritability, to rage. Users can become very aggressive and dangerous. For boys, their reproductive ability and sperm count are affected and in girls there is body and facial hair growth, and deepening of the voice. In both genders there is a loss of scalp hair.

Students who experience discrimination are at risk of experimenting with drugs, because they are at a disadvantage; they encounter further practices of exclusion and marginalization and cannot fit in the system. Children unconsciously work to create a world which mirrors their own internal wishes. They yearn for a response, even a negative one, in order to convince themselves that they really exist. Normally, teachers' reaction to their lack of success is overcome by feelings of rage, frustration and helplessness. They think the child is acting out in a dramatic

---

[49]   *Parade*, June 12, 2011.

way in order to provoke a response from them. Many children are misunderstood, misdiagnosed and prejudged by untrained and impatient teachers.

Teachers often wear the psychologist hat and use different strategies to keep students engaged in the room; they may move a disruptive student to sit alone, ask a student to calm down before rejoining the classroom, talk to a student about his/her behaviors. If a student has been labeled as being difficult, teachers typically expect that student to have challenging behaviors, including drug abuse. The expectations of others influence behavior. Some students are likely to live up to them. Every student is different and may have different needs when in an emotionally charged and confrontational classroom environment. Students' behaviors go across the ability range; they may become bored and therefore disruptive, or experiment with drugs. Anxious students may be held back by getting absorbed in one activity with no ability to change. This is especially a concern with minorities and culturally challenged children.

For some a teen's and adolescents' home can be an issue if the parents drink or use drugs. Parental substance abuse was predictive of adolescent substance abuse. Many adolescent alcoholics do not receive treatment. It was reported that students who were drinkers in seventh grade were most likely to have problems up to twelfth grade, with problems continuing into their twenties. Those problems ranged from a higher incidence of alcoholism; drug abuse such as cocaine and inhalants; predatory behaviors, violence, and drunk driving. Cocaine and inhalants have been linked to an increased risk for suicide among adolescents who had psychiatric disorders.

It is not certain how many teens abuse substances; according to National Institute of Drug Abuse (NIDA) there was about 23.5 million Americans age 12 and older who needed treatment in 2009. The National Organization of Adult, Children and Alcoholics reported 26.8 million children are alcoholics. Anyone can go to rehabilitation for substance abuse, but marijuana and other drugs can still circulate at the school and information about obtaining drugs can still be found on the Internet. Communities can help teens and adolescents by being supportive: give direction and hope, instead of guilt and shame which can fuel substance abuse. Addiction is very powerful; it allows self-medication as unwitting to cover abuse; feelings of anxiety and depression; and bulling at school. Teens and adolescents need sober friends, places and paths to go to and a plan to avoid the habit. Broken trust in teens takes time to rebuild; teens helping other teens to adjust could be instrumental in this process.

An intervention may or may not be relevant or effective for children from culturally different back grounds. There should be sufficient evidence or support for the effectiveness of a selected intervention, and preferably be a comprehensive, culturally-sensitive community prevention plan. Treatment should be tailored to cultural barriers such as mistrust, unfamiliarity with services, perceived culture competency and accommodation of teachers, and be aware to the lack of applicable skills and knowledge related to drugs.

When addressing cultural accommodation, modification must be made to treatment: adjusting components of the intervention to increase congruency with cultural norms. There must be consideration for the cultural and community context in which an intervention is implemented. There is a culture of addiction in modern societies which is much more prominent than in developing countries. An intervention has to target the identified problem by understanding factors that drive or contribute to changes in the outcomes. An intervention has to be appropriate for the particular population, culture context, and set of local circumstances.

The Role of Parents in Adjustment and Recovery from Addiction

A large body of theoretical and empirical work suggests that the quality of the parenting that children experience more strongly influences their adjustment than the type of family in which they are raised. The effects of family structure tend to be mediated through other aspects of the family environment and the parent-child relationship, including the parents' behavior. The characteristics of parents not only mediate the effects of family structure on the adjustment of children, but also moderate those effects. In the environment of low income single mothers there are monetary concerns for job stability, the source of income and control over household decisions; lack of financial support is likely to be integrated with lack of emotional support, mistrust of men and fear of domestic violence.

The offspring of violent fathers are already at a genetic risk for the development of behavior problems and mental disorders. These children have to be targeted for interventions which involve the entire family as early as possible. Despite the fact that fathers who engage in reckless and violent behavior make up a small proportion of fathers overall, they are responsible for a disproportional number of births. Historically, data on fathers have not been collected because mothers are considered the primary caretakers of their children and their parenting is considered the more important factor in children's adjustment. Fathers who engage in the most antisocial behaviors are generally the most difficult to interview. Some of these attempts suggest that these men are characterized by behaviors that may compromise their ability to be reliable sources of information. Parental presence is beneficial to children only when the parents are engaged in their activities.

Home, affection, and finances all play a role in adjustment and recovery of children. Critical issues of trust, love, and responsibility between children and parents may not be in balance; and issues of poor grades, arrests, lying, and dangerous accidents must be confronted. There should be a non-negotiable contract between parent and child, with consequences which are agreed upon. These may range from loss of social time away from the home, forfeiture of cell phones, withholding of allowances, or requiring jobs; withdrawal from extracurricular activities and sport teams, and removal from the school currently attended.

At a more restricted level there may be drug tests; teens/adolescents should be tested for drugs and alcohol randomly and unannounced, and be questioned about use. Family history matters in the overall assessment. Many teens attempt to escape the drama at home, the constant judging and negativity in school, by looking for insight, adventure, independence, and growth, and fall pray substance abuse. No friends or significant others should drink or use drugs in front of, or around, an adolescent in recovery. If there are alcoholics in the family, the family has to talk about this without rehashing or recriminating.

Treatment centers do not create recovery. They create a period of sobriety or abstinence from substances. While the addicted teen is adjusting in recovery, the family should reflect on new behaviors, new ways of communication and thinking. In the family, there should be a routine and requirements in place, with rules and expectations that must be met. It is very likely that attention-getting, through negative behavior, was learned and rewarded in the old family dynamic. The child was lost in a world of lies and self destruction—a very selfish world where the needs and demands were more important than anything else the world.

The family may get a phone call from their teenager at the treatment facility complaining of a variety of outrages or bad feelings, which is designed to justify leaving and coming home. The family should try not calling the facility during the first month and letting the center and its staff, along with the child, to do their job. However, family and mentors may send cards and letters of encouragement. Adjustment and recovery are bridges to the ability to trust the addict and let go, the resentment, anger, and doubt. The family must live the facts—there cannot be negotiation regarding relapse, dishonesty, theft, violence, or disappearance. The disease is not going away and it will always worsen if left unchecked. It is a product of who they are with, what they were doing, how they were doing in school, and how they were acting round others. Inpatient treatment is a logical step when outpatient treatment and local therapists have failed, because the environment and routine that the addiction has sustained itself in must be interrupted. The family itself may need a specific support group while they cope with treating their child, and may need to seek whatever counseling they can afford, by finding a therapist or counselor they can trust and talk.

The family cannot pray for miracles, it will need to work for them. A parent, a care giver, or counselor may come across as cold or unforgiving at times, but the truth is that what they are planning is the most forgiving effort there could ever be. Intervention is a profound act of love and hope in action. The family needs much support and empathizing with the truth of its own lonely struggle. Most family members with a lost child are incapable of rational thought and action. It is important to work as a team and not as individuals.

Outpatient programs must have a family group component. The earlier the intervention occurs, the healthier the children will be and the more apt they are to be mature in their decision making. The hardest part for parents is meaning what they say, following through, and recognizing the urgency called for in the face of crisis. Parental presence is beneficial to children only when they are engaged in their activities. A large body of theoretical and empirical work suggests that the quality of the parenting children experience more strongly influences their adjustment than the type of family in which they are raised.

Parents or other mentors should pay attention to their children's companions, music choices, art, and general moods, speech, and sleep patterns. There should be separation from peers and bad habits, and negative routines and pressures. There should be an establishment of structured, healthy alternatives that are free from major concerns and harmful influences.

The actual process in recovery is not better grades, a haircut, or getting back on the team. There should be only one requirement which is not success, nor a promise to succeed; for the child it is a desire to stop drinking and abusing drugs, and for the family it is love and acceptance. Everyone who is willing to try, who corrects behavior after each mistake, and who sincerely acknowledges error and supports common goals deserves another chance.[50] [51]

Invisible Addiction

Family members may seek to hide the consequences of addiction of other family members: such as by calling in sick in order to care for the affected individual who is ill from the effects of alcohol or drugs, or by lying to others about the reasons for the addicts' behavior. These actions are called enabling because they actively help addicts to avoid the consequences of their acts, and as a result they enable them to continue the addiction. This may partly explain why some codependent women always seem to end up in dysfunctional relationships with addicted men, and why some women appear to take on unhealthy or impaired men as "rehabilitation projects."

Invisible addiction also refers to groups of individuals who are perceived as overachievers, wealthy, and successful and who have the means to conceal their addiction. This includes those with a high status, such as elite celebrities and athletes. These individuals may experiment with a wide variety of addictive substances, because they may be inexperienced in handling the stress, the fame, and the influx of money. They may fear losing their identity, or "persona", to a competitor. As a maladaptive coping strategy, they sink into addiction, drugs and alcohol.

---

[50]   Finnigan, C. (2008) *When Enough is Enough*. New York: Penguin Group.

[51]   Gwinnell, E. (2006). *The A to Z of Addiction and Addictive Behaviors*. New York.

An Oregon congressman facing calls for his resignation from some of the state's largest newspapers said the addiction from which he suffered did not prevent him from doing his job. He blames the stresses of the campaign, and the responsibility and time involved in caring for his two children as reasons for his behavior—which included sending pictures of himself wearing a tiger costume to staff members. He later called these decisions "unprofessional and inappropriate" (Deseret News, February 27, 2011). The US Republican David Du said about this case: "If you do not stop drinking, don't brag about it, because people think that you have a problem . . . and if you ever go back to drinking people think you really have a problem." He was a political role model, newcomer when he was elected to congressman in 1998 and the first Chinese-American to serve in the US house. He has been seen as a leading voice on human rights abuse in China.

Another role-model, an Idaho senator, pleaded guilty to a charge of driving intoxicated.[52] He said that he began using alcohol as a misguided attempt to relieve stress. He kept his alcohol abuse hidden, drinking alone in his Washington D.C. apartment. Popular movie stars, musicians, fashion models and professional athletes are also reported often in the news and scrutinized for addiction, such as substance abuse, gambling, sex, eating disorders and autism.

Addiction in the Elderly

According to a survey conducted in 2012,[53] 8 to 9% of women and 4% of men reported severe psychological abuse (including engagement in illegal activities and using drugs) in childhood. More adults claim they faced psychological maltreatment in childhood than any other sort of abuse. Strong predictors in geriatric alcoholism and addiction are loneliness, grief or depression following the loss of a lifelong partner or a job, or isolation. Many alcoholic elderly suffer from vitamin and mineral deficiencies, especially of vitamin B12. This deficiency may present with symptoms of mental confusion, similar to what is seen with Alzheimer's disease. Elderly are more prone to developing most forms of cancer-related to alcoholism, especially esophageal cancer, and head, neck and liver cancer. If the alcoholic is a smoker the risk for lung cancer also increases. Adults who take morphine build up tolerance to the drug, but elderly people may be particularly sensitive to the side effects of morphine (e.g. hallucinations). Abandoning morphine, as the major pharmacotherapy for severe pain, is difficult and is a challenging task for the medical community.[54]

---

[52]   *Deseret News,* January 6, 2013.

[53]   *Deseret News,* August 5, 2012.

[54]   *Brain in the News,* May 2012.

Treating Drug Abuse and Quitting

Barriers to Treating Drug Abuse

Addiction and Self-Destruction

THE WRITER FYODOR Dostoyevsky and his followers pondered on the human penchant to pursue and endure suffering. In 1920, the father of psychoanalysis Sigmund Freud introduced the concept of the death instinct related to the aggressive drives to explain human destructiveness. Such formulations explain how much of the present psycho-negative stereotype of the addicted person as a pleasure seeker or as a self-destructive character originated from these early ideas. Understanding the destructive behavior associated with addiction is supported by a therapeutic approaches.

Today, the psycho-dynamic form of therapies effectively target and alter destructive behaviors by transforming patterns, of those that are predispose to addiction, in constructive ways, and building human connection. A competent clinician understands the core emotional and relationship dysfunctions when composing a comprehensive therapy. There is ample evidence that loneliness, depression, anxiety, and early trauma have an effect on the adoption of hedonistic behaviors and self-destructiveness seen in addicts.

In the early years of addiction treatment, there was actually very little agreement that addiction was an illness leading to self-destruction. Addiction was widely considered as a bad habit and an indication of a personal character flaw. Later, a comprehensive therapy provided a framework that allowed for societal functioning of addicts.[55]

Minor Consent Law, Labeling and Discrimination

Minor consent laws vary from state to state. Generally, parents hold the right to know about their children; however, some parents are dysfunctional and cause more harm when they know. In one survey, adolescents (10%) reported not visiting their healthcare providers in the previous year despite their wish to receive help because of fear that their parents would find out. Girls ages 12-17 (60%) reported that if their parents knew they would stop using health services and delay treatment.

There is also the stigma of labeling. Substance use disorders and addiction are recognized as impairment; this can and does, for many individuals, substantially limit their major life activities. For this reason, individuals who are in recovery from these conditions are individuals with a "disability" and are protected by federal law. This excludes those who currently engage in illegal use of drugs and are thus not protected under the non-discrimination laws. The limits on rights and opportunities due to drug convictions are as follows: public assistance and food stamps, student loans and financial aid, and having a driver's license. However, individuals may not be denied health services including drug rehabilitation based on their current illegal use of drugs.

Landlords and other housing providers cannot refuse to rent or sell homes to individuals in recovery. They may not discriminate in other ways in housing transactions based on disability. Addicts who feel discriminated may file a complaint with the Office of Civil Rights. The deadline for filing these complaints can be as soon as 180 days after the discriminatory act.

Discrimination against someone on the basis of his/her disability is illegal. Addicts in treatment or in recovery from substance use disorders are also protected from losing their jobs. All employees who are offered a position should be given the same exam. Employers may not deny a job or fire a person because s/he is in treatment or in recovery. Moreover, they must be provided with reasonable accommodation if the employee attends treatment.

Recovering employees should undergo medical examination only when doing so is job related and is justified by business necessity. Employers may not fire or

---

[55]   Khantzlan, E. J, & Albanese, M. J. (2008)

refuse to hire any job applicant or employee solely because a drug test reveals the presence of a lawfully used medication. The addicted employee has the right to take medical leave from the job if s/he needs it for substance abuse treatment. The Workforce Investment Act (WIA) provides financial assistance for job training and placement services for many addicts through the One Stop Career Center System.

Addiction and Learned Helplessness

According to the psychologist Albert Ellis (Rational Emotive Behavior Therapy), the primary cause of learned helplessness is the continual repetition of certain common irrational beliefs; needing to be loved, being successful, and pursuing money and happiness. Individuals who learn helplessness say to themselves: "I will never be loved, successful, have money, and/or happiness." Also, the individual believes that they will cause negative events to happen as part of their irrational belief. Depression occurs when the individual realizes that a different reality exists and when s/he makes internal stable and global attributions for it. Low self esteem is reflective of their views of a negative event as their own fault: "I caused my wife to leave me," "I caused my parents to get divorced," "I caused my father to become abusive," "I caused my son to get in trouble." This learned helplessness model is not a general theory of learning but instead applies to the cognitive processes associated with depression.

Learned helplessness refers to the tendency to give up any effort to control events in the environment. It was first observed in animals; when animals were exposed to uncontrollable events they subsequently did not try to escape these events, even when it was possible to do so. There are three aspects of self-control that increase the vulnerability for helplessness. These aspects are: self-monitoring–selectively attending to negative aspects of self control; self evaluation–making inaccurate internal attributions and comparing behaviors to standards that are excessively rigid and perfectionistic; and self-reinforcement–engaging in low rates of self-reward and high rates of self-punishment. In self-monitoring the individual records information about the frequency and conditions surrounding the negative thoughts and depressive episodes. In self-evaluation, the individual makes incorrect, biased and subjective irrational beliefs. In self reinforcement, the individual creates a negative, vicious cycle of their thoughts.

According to psychiatrist Aaron Beck's cognitive therapy, a person's cognitive schema may predispose the individual to depression and other disorders. In order to help people out of a destructive way of thinking, Socratic dialogue or guided discovery can be used; this involves asking questions that are designed to help the individual reach logical conclusions about the problem and its consequences. The "downward arrow" is the term used to question the evidence, "if so, then what"?

Attribution retraining focuses on altering the individual's perception and has been successfully used to treat depression, anxiety, and addiction. The techniques used are decatastrophizing, training away from negative mental imagery or creating positive mental imagery, and cognitive rehearsal. Thought-stopping is used when compulsive behaviors and addiction are in place. It has been used as part of the psychologist's Lynn Rehm's self-control therapy to treat depression and PTSD.

Addiction and Expectations

When expectations are not met, they produce mind and body tension and a sense of discontentment, damage, or devastation. Expectations could be: "my husband must not be so disrespectful"; "my wife must know what I need"; "I have to have my bedroom organized and clean daily"; "no one has the right to tell me what to do". Expectations trigger a fear-based reaction and heighten the sense of feeling threatened. Expectations that focus on others rather than on the self prevent individuals from thinking about their own character. However, a good husband, a spiritual acquaintance, or a dedicated wife can be excellent listeners when expectations are not met. The stronger the aversion was when expectations are not orderly fulfilled, the more likely the desired expectation was a requirement for the well-being of that individual.

In the course of therapy, the individual becomes aware of his/her perception and how it could be changed to bring peace. During therapy, individuals are given a hand mirror and are asked to look at themselves while jotting down on a blank piece of paper what comes into their mind about how they had these ingrained expectations. An individual comes home feeling tired and stressed. S/he is unable to regulate internal emotions and physiological expectations/reactions and may lash out at everyone else. These individuals are asked to find their most important personal qualities, and tune in to their body sensations, along with using compassionate and caring words to describe themselves.

Addiction and Automatism

Craving or drug hunger can be more compelling than almost any other need a human being can experience. The longer the struggle goes on, the harder it gets, and in the end control is lost. Over a period, something that started out in the realm of choice becomes involuntary (or automatic), and demands effort to control ("we were powerless over alcohol", AA). Loss of control is the result of having acquired something that has taken control for itself. We tend to think about it quantitatively rather than qualitatively—focusing on how much or how often the individual with addiction drinks or uses drugs rather than listening to what is experienced.

Using the drug again inevitably starts automatism and each time the addiction is reinforced—making automatism more efficient. Alcoholism or drug addiction cannot return to a casual drinking or drug use; proponents of this theory claim the addiction never goes away because automatism cannot be unlearned ("once an alcoholic is always an alcoholic", AA). The state of moderate casual drinking itself is not particularly dangerous; however, if the drinking is past this state, the individual becomes clumsy, uncoordinated, temporary disabled, and consequently endangers themselves. If s/he repeatedly puts him/herself in this dangerous condition, the brain begins to build up tolerance or resistance to the substance. A drug addict who is disoriented loses fair judgment; if s/he notices the curtains have caught fire, his/her mentality may be "who cares?" S/he may find the flames fascinating rather than getting him/herself to safety.

Newly abstinent individuals with alcoholism and addiction behave the way they feel without using substances to mask their personality characteristics. They may be irritable, depressed, untrusting, unloved and unloving. These types of personality characteristics might be caused by other issues such as oral fixation, impulsivity, dependency, depression, anxiety, and suppressed homosexuality. Research shows that many sociopaths become alcoholics, but they do not behave like sociopaths until after they developed alcoholism. When addiction is illegal, individuals spend a good deal of time and energy becoming experts in the predatory world. They develop characteristics typical of those with antisocial personality disorder. Lying, cheating, fighting, and acting on impulse become automatic behaviors. The 12-step program is, intentionally, not run by professionals but by recovering addicts and alcoholics themselves. The concept is that going to program meetings is like taking prescribed medicine, therefore professional treatment, with the prescription of drugs, and the 12-step programs are incompatible. Unfortunately, only 26% of individuals with addiction take their medications exactly as prescribed. For example, very few patients voluntarily take naltrexone for long periods of time. The idea that alcoholics have to be abstinent to begin recovery seems paradoxical because if they were able to stay sober, they would not be coming to treatment.

Understanding addiction and automatism require a balance between knowledge (information) and experience. A little knowledge may be dangerous but little understanding is even worse. An individual may relapse because s/he is short on knowledge and understanding on how to minimize the addiction. It seems the only difference between the type of addiction (gambling, eating, sex as sport, etc) is the cultural acceptability of the substance or activity involved

The whole idea of addiction as a curable condition is a result of not understanding automatism. Chemistry (medications/pills) may supply temporary relief from cravings, in the form of sedation, tranquilization, and even energy, but it still neglects understanding automatism, and does not develop courage and selflessness. Addicts remain with maladaptive coping mechanisms because no medicine, nor passively received treatment, can ever produce that understanding.

If an individual is abstinent, craving usually dies away on its own. Craving comes when patients are bored, lonely, angry, hurt, or want to party.

The therapist's impressions of the individual and the individual's description of his/her own experiences are inherently subjective and very difficult to quantify. A man who drinks only once a year, but each time he does he loses control and ends up in a self-destructive binge, is an alcoholic by qualitative standards. Relapsing again and again to automatic behaviors that end in trouble suggests an interfering mechanism. Treatment is difficult from social and cultural perspectives; individual variations among patients indicate the level of motivation, mental capacity, and physical health. The therapist must inquire why the patient is coming to treatment and how s/he was treated before. If the patient does not really want to get rid of his/her desire to drink, and instead wants to be able to drink like a non-alcoholic without the automatization (i.e., casually drink), then the drinking is still taking over his/her life. Those who continue to drink get worse and those who remain abstain do not. Among the most important factors are the therapist's personality characteristics: qualities such as warmth, genuineness, and capacity for nonjudgmental regard. Abstinence alone may be a form of self-denial and only recovery is the solution.

There are smokers who try to excuse themselves from the dangers and problems associated with addiction, by arguing that tobacco addiction does not lead to overdose, and unlike other drug addicts they are not in danger of getting HIV or hepatitis, being arrested for stealing or prostitution. A strictly medical treatment of addiction may convey long term benefits. Medications such as methadone and buprenorphine eliminate cravings for heroin, morphine, and oxycodone, they are longer-acting drugs of the same kind.

Addiction and Withdrawal Symptoms

Withdrawal symptoms of addiction vary according to the nature of the addiction: from mood disturbances such as anxiety, depression, agitation, irritability, and restlessness to physical symptoms such as chills, shaking, profuse sweating, and abdominal pain. Rebalancing the body and brain biochemistry makes it possible for the addict to address the behavioral, emotional, and spiritual aspects of their addiction and endure the withdrawal symptoms. Until the mid-eighties, addiction treatment attracted the attention of research studies on recidivism. Despite the fact that the life circumstances of addicts had dramatically improved, quitting alcohol had left them with depression and anxiety. Some of them actually felt worse in recovery than they had felt while they were using substances. Substance abuse masks emotional pain but residents of inpatient programs receive extensive therapy to explain underlying psychological issues.

The mid-eighties brought the crack cocaine epidemic, accompanied with a high relapse rate. Treatment for addiction to crack cocaine failed due to the lack of integration of amino acids in the diets of patients. A corrective diet has also helped with marijuana, alcohol, and other stimulant addictions. In cases where marijuana was used by an individual as an anesthetic to alleviate pain, the pain returned if the individual ate something to which s/he was allergic. Individuals are often allergic to the drug or substance they are addicted to, which makes withdrawal even more painful. Any substance under the sun, including sunlight itself, can cause an allergic reaction. An allergy to vitamin B can prevent the absorption of nutrients and produce cravings; for example, some individuals crave smoking because they need the niacin. Consumption of certain foods can also be dangerous. Foods that contain artificial sweeteners, additives, and coloring contain chemicals which could be neurotoxic.

The electromagnetic field of toxins, such as mercury and types of metal, impairs the blood flow inside the brain. Research has found a connection between energy toxins and withdrawal. Disturbances in the energy field often result from energy toxins or allergy sensitivity and intolerance. Heavy metals create interference on both physical and electromagnetic levels and are a common factor in addiction. The body, which is the environment for the energetic levels, is subjected to toxic buildup and requires cleansing and restoration to good health. There is a need to cleanse the energy field from toxins that are interfering with the physical, emotional and spiritual health of the individual. A holistic integrated therapy is likely to be more effective than just talking therapy. A therapist who looks at the development of disharmony with the substance underneath can sometimes uncover the root of many addictions and causes of relapse (such as abuse and withdrawal that can change the user's energy level).

Special Cases: Addiction and Autism
(see Appendix A for more information)

One of the main barriers in trying to cure addiction is in aiding those from challenging populations due to their behaviorally unique attributions and brain chemistry. Since the prevalence of autism seems to be on the rise, much attention has been given to finding remedies to stop addiction which is associated with this condition. Individuals with autism have larger brains which are overdeveloped and oversensitive. Their brains have dense neural wiring which enables them to remember details, and they become easily oversaturated. In autism, there is a diminuend activity in the left brain hemisphere and increased activity in the right hemisphere. Therefore these individuals have to think less with the right hemisphere. Improving a hemisphere which is in charge of language, without also developing spatial learning and emotional content, creates a problem.

Individuals with autism require more logical, sequential and rhythmical skills, which includes balancing their movements which are asymmetrical. Eye contact is difficult, especially for those who cannot process what they are seeing at the same time that they are processing what they are hearing. Individuals with autism cannot understand feelings and beliefs; they cannot reason, empathize, or connect with other people. There is a deficiency in reflecting mirror neurons, which only allows for imitation of expression.

Individuals with autism are sensitive; for example, they may cry listening to certain types of music. The background sound and melody improve their communication and emotional reaction. However, loud music can be stressful. Singing is recommended for those with autism; it is like learning a new language. However, sensory overload from sound, light or the combination of both can prevent them from 'feeling' their body. Such sensory overload may result in the individual being unable to keep their clothes on even when it is chilly outside, because everything feels like sandpaper on the skin. Trying to act socially in gatherings such as meeting or parties is really difficult as they are overwhelmed with the light, the crowd and the background noises that are usually present in these situations.

Ways which have been normally used to help individuals who have sensitivities to light and sound are: wearing a baseball cap or hat with a brim and sunglasses to help with keeping bright lights out of the eyes in brightly lit environments; desensitization, for example, by going into an overly-lit store a few minutes for the first time and then increasing the time spent in the store thereafter; wearing headphones with music or ones that are noise-cancelling in a noisy environment. These are some of the barriers to consider when treating individuals with autism when they exhibit particular personality traits, moods, and anxiety or impulse control disorders.

Auditory integration therapies require individuals to wear headphones and listen to modulated sounds and music, with certain frequencies filtered out. Vision therapy consists of a combination of exercises and lenses, which is effective in helping process incoming information correctly. Occupational therapy helps individuals meet goals in areas of everyday life that are important to them, and helps with proprioceptive and vestibular dysfunctions.

Sensory Integration Therapy targets the way the brain organizes sensations and input received in order to better engage in the environment. Rocking, for instance, stimulates the vestibular system connected to the cerebellum and provides the brain's wiring mechanism. Movement is a good thing—it wires the brain. It is called "a self-regulatory behavior". Children do it to both provide stimulation to their nervous systems and to calm themselves. However, it becomes a debilitating sensory addiction, engagement or interaction with an autistic child which requires an immediate response. All babies are hedonic in the way they seek pleasure, and are not very different than what is seen in individuals with autism, who are stuck at this stage and unable to delay gratification. Babies and individuals with autism are self-centered and are addicted to sensory play and repeated movement (touch, suck, rock). Sensory play and excessive repetitive movement ("known as the runners high"), produce beta-endorphins which are associated with changes in mood and pain thresholds.

Conditioning and desensitization can start early–when children refuse to allow their hair cut, brushed, or shampooed because their scalp is too sensitive and it feels extremely painful to have any kind of touch. The same applies to brushing teeth and sensitive gums. These individuals exhibit sensory dysfunction in the form of hypo-deep tactility. This puts them at risk of hurting themselves and/or others, exhibiting improper behaviors without their awareness. An inappropriate behavior would be throwing themselves on the floor at the signs of a temper tantrum, wetting the pants in a public area, becoming upset and screaming. They may act in pain every time they are picked up because they are sensitive to touch.

Addiction to sensory play stems from two main sources: producing endorphins (endogenous morphine) which influences mood and pain perception, and seeking good feelings and avoiding painful withdrawal symptoms. Children with autism are attracted to emotional thrills, danger, fear, or rage, and self-comforting and self-hypnosis behaviors. The addicted brain learns and craves those extreme experiences again. The emotional arousal which comes with the addiction is dependent on the individual's mental development. Since the child interacts much better with videos, computer games, and TV animated features than with a live person, important developmental skills are necessary for the child to initiate, develop, and maintain relationships.

When a child is born s/he learns about the world by using his/her senses. The child learns about the world by putting everything in their mouths, grabbing objects in their fingers, and looking at mobiles hanging over the crib. They learn to recognize the sound of their mother's and other's voices in order to make meaning of the world around. If these images, smells, flavors and noises are not working properly and are not in synchrony, the child acquires a distorted view of the world and of themselves. The Sensory Processing Disorder is a neurological disorder that causes difficulties with processing information from the five senses–vision, auditory, touch, olfaction, and taste–as well as from the sense of movement (vestibular system), and/or the positional sense (proprioception). Information is processed by the brain in an unusual way that causes distress, discomfort, and confusion. Sensory integration therapies include: auditory, vision, and occupational.

People may experience a sensory processing disorder, but do not show any diagnostic signs of autism. However, sensory processing–making sense of the world–is what most adults on the autism spectrum conveyed as the most frustrating area they struggled with as children. It impacted every aspect of their lives–relationships, communication, self-awareness, and safety. Many adults who struggle with addiction are child-like in their ability to be in relationships with other people.

Autism as a sensory disorder, rather than a psychiatric diagnosis, can be viewed as a labyrinth of addiction. Cravings for sugar, milk and gluten products may cause behavioral and mental interference and disorganization. Individuals with autism cannot metabolize those substances properly, which makes them toxic in their bodies and brains. In addition, most individuals on the Autism Spectrum who are Salicylate intolerant become addicted to food substances that are high in Salicylates and Phenols. Salicylates are derivatives of salicylic acid that occur naturally in plants and serve as a natural immune hormone and preservative, protecting the plants against diseases, insects, fungi, and harmful bacteria. Salicylates can also be found in many medications, perfumes and preservatives. Both natural and synthetic salicylates can cause health problems in anyone when consumed in large doses, but for those who are salicylate intolerance, even small doses of salicylate can cause adverse reactions.

Prevalent approaches to cure this addiction include Biomedical Interventions in the form of diets and supplements. Behavioral conditioning is a very simplistic way of treating those with sensory disorders that are attached to autism. It is derived from classical conditioning to explain a variety of human responses from emotional reactions and attitudes to addiction. Addiction can be treated and cured with a high-order conditioning. When a second neutral stimulus is repeatedly paired with a previously conditioned stimulus (smell/flavor of food high in sallcylates and phenols), the second neutral stimulus eventually produces a conditioned response (eating the healthy food).

Desensitization is a technique that is also used in a way that a relaxing image is paired with the presentation of items in an anxiety hierarchy, beginning with the least anxiety-evoking item. Interventions based on aversive counter conditioning are: in-vivo aversion therapy and covert sensitization. The target behavior that the therapist wants to eliminate from the patient is paired with an aversive stimulus. Aversion therapy is more effective when it is administered in conjunction with other treatments. Multiple cumulative stimuli involve repetitive patterns and emotional extremes. Covert sensitization is used to eliminate a maladaptive behavior by implanting an imagination of an aversive stimulus when an individual begins to engage in a maladaptive behavior. Conditioning via visualization (not conceptualization) and with concrete examples seems to work the best.

Autism is more than an information processing disorder; social skill training is used to improve communication, assertiveness, problem-solving, and other socially adaptive skills. It is classified as a type of behavior therapy that incorporates techniques derived from operant and classical conditioning as well as from social learning theory. Specific techniques include: modeling, coaching, behavioral rehearsal, feedback, reinforcement, and homework assignment. Social skill training is an effective intervention for: reducing symptoms, decreasing the risk for relapse, and improving social adjustment. It helps reduce depression when used as part of multimodal treatment approach. There is evidence-based research of the mind on patients with schizophrenia and improvement of behavior among children with conduct who suffered trauma.

Addiction and various co-occurring disorders often interfere with the development of the mind's structure, which has lead some researchers to look at trauma therapy for autism. Many of those who struggle with addiction also wrestle with untreated underlying trauma (Stanley Greenspan, Appendix A). Long-term success in dealing with addiction necessitates replacing unhealthy relationships to objects with healthy relationships to people. These skills are critical in relating to others in many contexts: intimate relationships, child rearing, work environments, and marriage. They may never be developed due to trauma or time spent with addictions. Creating these healthy relationships can be an especially difficult hurdle for those with autism

Therapeutic Solutions

Medication-assisted treatment follows a medical assessment and a comprehensive assessment to determine the patient's motivation. Prior to treatment there is an observation of the patient's allergic reaction and determining if the patient has any cardiac abnormalities. Monitoring drug use and prenatal care is critical for those who are on medication assisted treatment. A large percentage of pregnant women continue to use substances that are harmful to maternal and fetal health (alcohol, heroin, cocaine, barbiturates, and tranquilizers). All patients have to pass four phases in treatment.

In the acute phase of detoxification, the goals are: to eliminate withdrawal symptoms and opioid craving, abstain from illicit opioid use, comply with treatment medication regimen, conform to drug tests, learn about drug and medication interaction risks, avoid high risk situations for relapse, actively engage in recovery, complete medical and health follow up assessments, and finish a treatment plan.

In the rehabilitation phase, there should be increased efforts to promote patients' participation in constructive activities such as employment, education, vocational training, child rearing, homemaking and volunteer work. This phase may offer a support group to help patients discontinue alcohol and prescription drug abuse as well as illicit-drug use, and acquire coping skills and relapse-trigger awareness. The goal in this phase is to empower patients to cope with major life problems by accepting increased responsibility.

In the tapering and readjustment phase, the goals are: to re-educate and eliminate long-term use of the medications, increase self-sufficiency, maintain a balanced lifestyle and function well without medications. Patients have a good prognosis if they: work on making lifestyle changes to decrease the need for drugs, recognize relapse warning signs, avoid people and situations that might trigger use, develop positive coping methods, and participate in healthy, rewarding activities as alternatives to drug use. Although, medication-assisted treatment frees the addict from thinking about the drug and reduces problems of withdrawal or craving, psychotherapy induces feelings of self-worth.

Patients are likely to retain treatment if the admission process is simplified, and if attention is given to their financial needs. If the staff is knowledgeable, and has a positive attitude and confidence about the efficacy of the program, patients are likely to adopt this attitude. Therapists who view addiction as biologically driven alone are misinformed. Philosophy for treatment should derive from a holistic social science approach. Passion, hard work, and a calling to serve can make a difference in the patient's life. Some patients are often cynical about the value of the therapeutic intervention and this cynicism may come from ignorance.

Functional Behavioral Analysis

Functional behavioral analysis is conducted to determine the purpose of the behavior and identify a more desirable substitute behavior that serves the same purpose. For example, a school psychologist might conduct an analysis to identify the purpose of a student's inattentive and disruptive behaviors; the student may act that way to imitate his/her parents.

We tend to imitate models of power and admiration; models of higher status, prestige and expertise. According to the observational and social learning theory, the characteristics of the model are likely to be from the same culture, ethnicity, environment, and to be deemed similar to the observer's own characteristics. Self-efficacy, a central concept in psychologist Albert Bandura's theory, is instrumental in recovery; it refers to the individual's beliefs about his/her ability to perform the behavior, and achieve the task and the goal. Bandura has defined self-efficacy as one's belief in one's ability to succeed in specific situations. One's sense of self-efficacy can play a major role in how one approaches goals, tasks, and challenges. The theory of self-efficacy lies at the center of Bandura's social cognitive theory, which emphasizes the role of observational learning and social experience in the development of personality. The main concept in social cognitive theory is that an individual's actions and reactions, including social behaviors and cognitive processes, in almost every situation are influenced by the actions that individual has observed in others. The relationship between the individual's environment, overt behaviors, and cognitive, affective and other personal characteristics is considered to be reciprocal determinism. Several strategies are used to help the individual adopt a positive-problem solving orientation and a rational problem-solving style. These include: psycho-education, guided discussion, role playing, and homework assignment.

Self-management procedures are an umbrella for a variety of strategies which emphasize the individual's responsibility for modifying his/her behaviors. These procedures add self-monitoring, to the self-instruction and to thought stopping. An educational procedure helps the client understand his/her dysfunctional self-control behaviors and cognitive responses are stress inoculated. The individual learns and rehearses a variety of coping skills that include: direct-action (relaxation, pleasant imagery, arranging escape routes) and cognitive techniques (replacing negative self-statements with coping self-statements).

Conditioning as a Treatment

The environment and settings (place, friends, particular location, certain rituals, etc.) associated with the substance are conditioned stimuli. This can also be as simple as craving the substance. Relapse is likely to occur when facing "refresher trials" which are difficult to resist. Refresher trials are when an addict remains an addict when s/he goes back to the same environment and setting, facing those temptation cues.

Addiction can be treated and re-cured with a high-order conditioning. When a second neutral stimulus is repeatedly paired with a previously conditioned stimulus, the second neutral stimulus eventually produces a conditioned response. For example, when alcohol is paired with images of relaxations to relieve pain, the alcohol becomes the conditioned response for emotional pain. Recovery fails if there is blocking, or submission of redundant information. When the addiction cue is stronger than the recovery cue ("just one more cigarette or drink will not kill me"), the short term gratification overpowers the long term consequences of dying and delays recovery. According to the American psychologist John Watson, threat and trauma to an addict's existence and enforcing external reinforcements inhibit recovery. This theory addresses the establishment of phobia and stimulus generalization.

Interventions based on counter-conditioning, according to Joseph Wolpe's behavioral therapy, use incompatible response to eliminate stress associated with certain experiences (for instance, using relaxation techniques instead of alcohol, cigarettes, and opiates). During relaxation training the therapist teaches the addict to use a technique that produces a state of relaxation. Progressive relaxation is a commonly used technique that involves systematically tensing and relaxing all of the body's major muscle groups. It often begins with a standard cue such as taking a deep breath or saying "I am relaxed." Alternatively, the addict may imagine a relaxing scene such as lying on the beach.

Interventions based on aversive counter-conditioning are used to eliminate a maladaptive behavior by having the addict imagine an aversive stimulus when they begin to imagine engaging in the maladaptive behavior. The target behavior is paired with an aversive stimulus. Aversion therapy is more effective when it is supplemented by "booster sessions" or is administered in conjunction with another therapy. Covert sensitization is used to eliminate a maladaptive behavior by having the addicts imagine an aversive stimulus when they begin to imagine engaging in the maladaptive behavior

For instance, to reduce cigarette smoking, the therapist may instruct the addict to imagine smoking a cigarette and then visualize becoming nauseated by the taste, followed by engaging in alternative behaviors (e.g. envisioning relief scenes of pleasant sensations). A similar technique that is frequently used to treat alcohol and drug addictions is in-vivo aversion therapy. The therapist instructs the addict to imagine drinking alcohol, then throwing up which is then substituted with soothing feelings. A photo of a sick liver as a result of drinking alcohol or a strong alcoholic odor will result in nausea.

Interventions based on classical extinction expose the addict to the conditioned stimulus (alcohol, drug, cigarettes) without the unconditioned stimulus (anxiety, stress, pain). They inhibit the usual avoidance response (drinking, smoking, using the substance) in order to extinguish the conditioned response. When the individual is exposed to the distressing stimulus and is prevented from responding in their usual way by eliminating the availability of the substance, s/he has to face the problem and deal with it, rather than avoiding and trying to forget. Implosive theory is essentially the same—it is conducted in the imagination with the only difference being that it involves presenting the feared stimulus vividly enough so as to arouse high levels of anxiety. Classical extinction relies heavily on group support to provide the necessary support and emotional strengthen to sustain abstinence.

In order to desensitize addiction, an individual's imagination must be utilized. Relaxation is paired with the presentation of items in the anxiety hierarchy beginning with the least anxiety-evoking item. The therapist instructs the patient to relax using the relaxation techniques the client learned during the first stage of treatment. Once the client is relaxed, the therapist instructs him/her to imagine the appropriate anxiety hierarchy item. The addict signals the therapist whenever s/he feels anxious, and the therapist helps the addict reestablish a state of relaxation before the next item in the hierarchy is presented. This process is repeated until the addict is able to imagine the most anxiety arousing item without experiencing stress or anxiety.

Social skill intervention is used to improve communication, assertiveness, problem-solving, and other socially adaptive skills. It is classified as a type of behavioral therapy that incorporates techniques derived from operant and classical conditioning and social learning theory. Specific techniques include: modeling, coaching, behavioral rehearsal, feedback, reinforcement, and homework assignment. Social skill training is an effective intervention for reducing symptoms, decreasing the risk for relapse, and improving social adjustment. It helps reduce depression when used as part of a multimodal treatment approach. There is evidence-based research on the effectiveness of this invention on patients with schizophrenia and improvement of behavior among children with conduct problems.

Reinforcements

Brain researchers looked at brain rhythms in a region at the very bottom of the basal ganglia known as the ventral striatum. According to Brain in the News,[56] patterns of electrical activity in part of the brain known as the basal ganglia are critical for habit information. The area which is necessary for responding to pain and pleasure is also highly involved in addiction, and in learning a new behavior. The high frequency activity in the output neurons of the ventral striatum sends messages to the rest of the brain directing it to learn a new behavior. Identifying and controlling such neurons might offer a new way to help combat addiction.

Addicts can be conditioned to do things which are rewarding, even activities that are initially difficult, painful or awkward. They can be rewarded for their hard work, diligence or thoughtfulness by being given praise, increasing their self-esteem, achieving high grades at school or by recognition, pay increase or promotion at their jobs, affection, and love. Addicts can be conditioned to learn to make long-term plans, defer gratifications, and accommodate their own desires.

Unfortunately, drug taking is also self-reinforcing, and the payoff is the drug experience itself. This kind of reinforcement is the "recipe" for psychological dependence, because the drug user is convinced that the effects of the drug are necessary for his/her function. Addiction has long been considered a response to the loss of status and boredom. The concentration of drug abuse in the inner city may reflect high rates of unemployment. Among these addicts there can be found many enablers; these are denoted individuals who contribute to the addiction or another abuse, most often passively.

Regrettably, an enabler is someone in the environment who forgives and tolerates compulsive drug use, lends money and overlooks outrageous behavior. An enabler fails to confront the abuse and hopes the symptoms s/he observes will go away in time. However, they may not understand that abusers are not dependable and irresponsible because of their preoccupation with drugs. Physical dependency develops when body cells are changed by constant exposure to the drug, that the user becomes incapable of functioning properly when deprived if the substance. For instance, a coffee drinker with a daily, multi-cup habit will suffer headaches if abruptly deprived of coffee. Likewise, an opiate addict will suffer stress due to drug deprivation.

Understanding stress and opiate addiction is based upon conditioning and reinforcements. Opiate induced euphoria is mediated via endogenous opioid peptide systems in the brain to constitute a positive reinforcer which makes repeated use more likely even before physical dependence and tolerance develop. At that point, withdrawal symptoms arise, becoming a negative reinforcer, and also motivates the addicts to seek and use opiates more frequently. It is the interplay between the

---

[56] *Brain in the News,* October, 2011.

positive reinforcer of opiate-induced euphoria and the negative reinforcer of opiate withdrawal that forms the strong underpinnings of addiction. The strength of this interplay between positive and negative reinforcers (or mood states) is underscored by the hazards that addicts grow to tolerate as part of their addictive lifestyle. The development of depression in an opiate addict can be viewed as another negative reinforcer of continued opiate use. Depressed opiate addicts may self-medicate depressive symptoms with opiates to relieve stress and feel euphoria.

Addicts may be subjected to trials and errors before they become addicts and the desired effect of their drug use is reached via instrumental learning. According to the Law of Effect by American psychologist Ted Thorndike, any response that is followed by a satisfying state of affairs is unlikely to be repeated while any act that results in an annoying state of affairs is likely to be repeated. Positive reinforcements are the expectations from the drug for rewarding consequences; negative reinforcements are the withdrawal effects which foster the behavior or the addiction. The addict attempts to eliminate the withdrawal symptoms through negative reinforcements. When the substance is suddenly unavailable the individual may go to extremes and use a certain behavior as a trade off to get it (e.g. prostitution). In this vulnerable state it gets out of control, s/he is prone to being abused, exploited, taken advantage of, and held deprived from primary necessities such as food and shelter. The addict may try to escape the pain and discomfort by continuing using the drugs.

The matching law to Thorndike's implies that correspondence to one of two or more alternatives to drug use and withdrawal depends on the frequency of reinforcement for that behavior. A combination of therapies that compose an eclectic comprehensive approach fosters a stronger resilient behavior to avoid the drug. A superstitious competing behavior may disturb this process if this becomes an old ritual or an obsessive-compulsive behavior. This suspicious behavior may seem to the addict detrimental to survival because it suppressed the pain and with it the suffering. Superstitious behavior is a distorted perception and certainly not a solution to the problem.

In the two factor learning theory, avoidance conditioning takes into consideration the physiological as well as the psychological conditions. Through escape and avoidance conditioning, addicts may flee from punishment and other sanctions. Avoidance behaviors and maladaptive coping mechanisms are learned during childhood and may represent conflicts related to sexual or aggressive impulses.

Drugs require stimulus control and control cues to prevent relapse. In order to increase a positive change by reinforcement, a contingent relationship between the target behavior and the positive reinforcer must follow immediately and with the schedule of reinforcement, otherwise superstitious behavior could occur. The magnitude of verbal clarification and verbal or physical prompts facilitate the acquisition of a new behavior. An individual does not relapse if the benefits and outcomes of abstinence outweigh the short term reward–the pleasure principle of the drug.

The Premack principle is used to increase the amount of abstinence by providing, for instance, assistance with financial resources, employment, and family and social services. Contingency contracts define the addicted behavior that is to be substituted, and the rewards and punishments that will follow. It is an application of contingency management that involves a formal written agreement between the therapist and an addict, or a parent and a child. Behavioral change may be required by one or all parties involved with the contract. A contingency contract between a therapist and an addict would require behavior change by the client only, while a contract between spouses would likely require change by both parties. Contingency contracts are most effective when the person whose behavior is to be modified actively participates in the development of the contract.

According to Stuart and Lott,[57] the contract must be explicit in defining what each party will receive as a result of meeting the responsibilities. The behaviors included in the contract must be capable of being monitored. A record-keeping system would be beneficial to provide constant feedback about the frequency of the target behaviors and the delivery of reinforcers. The contract also should have definitions of bonuses for consistent compliance with the terms of the contract. A list of sanctions for failure to meet the terms of the contract should be defined as well.

A common reinforcement practice in addiction treatment in order to increase positive change is a token economy. It takes place in structured environments because token economy is easier to control. Desirable behaviors are increased by reinforcing them with tokens or other generalized secondary reinforcers. These can be exchanged for desired items, activities, and other primary reinforcers. The undesirable behaviors are decreased by withholding or removing tokens following those behaviors. Token economies are associated with several advantages: they permit an immediate delivery of reinforcement and can be tailored to meet individual needs by allowing the individual to select their own incentives. They are also less susceptible than primary reinforcers to satiation because tokens can be exchanged for a variety of reinforcers in order to make the individual feel confident, relaxed, and happy.

Punishments

Punishments will decrease the addict's behavior, but punishment, such as incarceration, may fail because of low intensity and irremovability of all positive reinforcements. Reprimands can act as positive reinforcers and actually increase

57   Stuart, L. (1972). *Cognitive Behavior Therapy.* Hoboken, NJ: Wiley

the target behavior. The effects of verbal reprimands are likely to be temporary and inconsistent if they are not followed by other consequences. Punishment must be immediate, consistent, and intense. Initially administrating punishment in a weak form and then gradually increasing its intensity increases the likelihood of habituation which occurs when a punishment loses its effectiveness extinction is a preferable form than punishment to treat addiction.

Addictive behavior can be made extinct by withholding reinforcements from a previously reinforced response in order to eliminate or decrease the addiction. Extinction can be a slow frustrating process because it is often difficult to identify and consistently withhold all sources of reinforcement. Extinction is more rapid when the behavior has been reinforced on a continuous schedule than on an intermittent schedule. The longer the duration of the previous reinforcement the more resistant the extinction of the behavior is. Extinction is most successful when it is used in conjunction with reinforcements for alternative behaviors. This supports substituting the use of drugs with stress relaxation techniques and alternative social activities (e.g. dance, bowling, and recreation).

Overcorrection is another form which can be used in conjunction with extinction. It often includes providing verbal instructions that require constant supervision. When the individual corrects any negative effects of the behavior, it is called restitution. It requires the individual to practice more appropriate behavior (or positive behavior). Negative practices (e.g. alcohol or drug intoxication) require the individual to deliberately repeat the undesirable behavior to the point that it becomes aversive. Overcorrection can be problematic because it may elicit avoidant, resistant, or aggressive behavior. It eliminates habits and behaviors that the individual has not been able to control. Sometimes response cost is used instead as a strategy of negative punishment because it involves removing a specific behavior by taking away something meaningful, like imposing fines. This technique works particularly with sociopaths because they do not respect and do not conform to social norms and the law.

Self-Help Therapy

Recovered addicts have to avoid cues associated with drugs, and can do this by learning about toxic effects, drug fatalities, drug-induced psychoses, or other horrors which would help weaken their condition. It helps when they talk to themselves and practice self-restraint. *Controlled self-talk* can contradict negative thinking, self-doubts, and excuses. Self restraining imposes a delay on any decision regarding temptation. It lets the recovered addict consider the consequences of the actions in order to make a more logical decision and take control over the addiction. Three variables determine how much control a user is able to exercise over addiction:

the nature of the drug, the user's personality and attitudes about drug use, and the physical site and social framework within which drug use occurs.

Over-conditioning creates an aversion to the response, and *covert over-conditioning* asks the individuals to imagine decidedly unpleasant consequences for use of a drug. *Behavior modification* attacks the conditioned response that is responsible for compulsive drug abuse. It desensitizes users by weakening the stimulus–the trigger mechanism of the conditioned response. Modification types include relaxation techniques and hypnoses. *Hypnosis* provides decidedly unpleasant consequences for drug taking. Hypnosis has provided substitute gratification for detoxification, allowing addicts to re-experience a "good trip" from a satisfying drug reaction and relieve some depression and joylessness that accompany withdrawal.

Transcendental meditation helps deal with tension. *Electrotherapy* is a technique that resembles and is based upon the use of *acupuncture,* but with added electrical stimulation. *Electromyography* helps relieve distress and withdrawal, and enables the individual to loosen tightened muscles. *Exercise* is a means of expending energy and relieving feelings of tension and anxiety. Exercise such as hiking, biking, and running, or taking part in excursions and risk-taking activities (such as rock climbing, and water canoeing) build confidence and expand social contacts. Mood levels can be affected by poor diet, overweight and lack of exercise. Cooking, photography, signing up for college or graduate studies, joining a theatre group or a choral society are considered boosting, mood-relief therapies.

The *cue-exposure strategy* is another useful technique to plan a week in advance; the patient considers what s/he needs to enjoy life, and whether the demands are reasonable and appropriate. Drug users tend to think of themselves as relatively helpless individuals. They feel guilty, embarrassed, and become easily manipulated and controlled. Consequently, users are generally angry and respond to legitimate concerns with hostility and a desire to use drugs again. Cue-exposure helps get the individual back on track, focused on the task, and understand what they want to accomplish. It also helps avoid distortions and negative influences.

Antagonist therapy also attempts to reverse the process of reinforcement. Antagonists work by moving receptor sites in the brain in a way that the drug of abuse cannot make a connection. Sometimes therapists recommend biofeedback. In *biofeedback* patients can learn to control their body response by observing what actions alter the tone of the display. Stimulus control and biofeedback are based on operant conditioning. A number of studies have found that relaxation training (e.g. autogenic training) is as effective as biofeedback.

In addition to self-help therapy, therapists offer enhancing techniques. *Contingency management* is suggested when the desirable behavior is bought with rewards. Should addicts violate the contract, the therapist will mail letters they wrote at the time they signed the contract. These letters contain confessions of drug use and they can go to employers, professional associations, licensing boards, families, and newspapers.

Acupuncture and Flower Essence Therapies

Research has shown that acupuncture produces good results when used during detoxification and as an initial treatment for heroin or cocaine addiction. Addicts may initially come for treatment for a skin condition, neck pain or headaches, and in the course of treatments they become motivated to deal with their substance problems. Effective treatment must go further than reducing cravings however. To address the root of the problem there are a set of behaviors that go with the use of substances. If the patient fails it is usually because s/he is unable to make the behavioral, psychological, and lifestyle changes necessary to end the addiction.

Flower essence therapy is the practice of using flower essences to experience emotional harmony and spiritual well-being. It provides a language that helps understand the inner world and the ways in which one responds to life and life's situations. Flower essences promote a return to health on all levels by addressing underlying psycho-spiritual issues and promoting energetic shifts in the mind and emotions. In flower essence therapy, the nature of pain is identified. For example, pain in alcoholism is most often a result of loneliness. These individuals need help dealing with their emotions and overwhelming anxiety. Instead of expressing their anger, they normally turn to drugs and alcohol.

Yerba Santa, also known as holy herb, is used to treat lung conditions and is recommended for treating physical and emotional states. The patterns of imbalance it cures affect these constricted feelings and deeply repressed emotions. Flower essence therapy can work on deep layers and can move people out of addiction to a path of enlightenment and to feeling better. A marijuana patient said that when he felt the hole in his soul, he took his flower essences a little more frequently, and gradually, the empty feelings subsided.

Faith-based approaches

The transformative power of faith can be central in reducing addiction. Faith-based programs have helped prisoners incorporate education and mentoring into their treatment. The faith factors are linked to inmate adjustment and to reductions in the likelihood of arrest following release from prison. Faith-based approaches are a new crime-fighting strategy targeted to communities facing crime-related challenges. The data and results to test the efficacy of the program are very limited because church leaders usually say they do not need academic research to validate their work: "we answer to God, not to researchers . . . we already know our programs are effective."

Quitting

Awakening

The first step in quitting addiction is awakening. Something happens in the life of the addict, which has an enormous impact, and causes a change in the individual's perception. During awakening the individual identifies the differences from the type of fear that keeps one safe and the fear that holds one back from reporting abuse, seeking help, and terminating harmful relationships. Awakening teaches a balance between power and compassion, fierceness and kindness. However, there are negative consequences associated with awakening: a spouse leaving, incarceration, loss of custody, problems at work, and DUI.

Addicts may desperately want to get rid of the addiction, but may not believe that it is possible to recover. They may be fearful of giving up the option of "getting high" because of painful inner conflicts or past trauma. The better an addict is able to tolerate the negative feelings the more they are able to experience contentment, which draws the line between addicts slipping and addict being successful at overcoming their addiction. A spouse can help (as much as sabotage) the awakening process. A spouse may try to mold his/her partner into a person s/he wants him/her to be, which may result in trauma, abuse and manipulation.

Some interventions and court mandated treatments are based on the premise that the addict cannot awake from the illness and therefore is not able to make rational choices. These programs for addicted individuals are highly confrontational and structured and do no substitute for group support. During awakening there are often revived interests in spiritual, religious, or in civic activities.

Effective Therapy

The second step in quitting addiction is finding an effective therapist. A prevailing view of substance abuse as a disease model of addiction was supported by both the National Institute of Drug Abuse and Alcoholics Anonymous. The model attributed addiction largely to changes in brain structure and function. Health experts recommend professional treatment and complete abstinence and do not believe in successful recovery without professional help. However there have been cases where individuals did not need to seek professional help to overcome addiction. During the Vietnam War, the majority of soldiers who became addicted to narcotics later stopped using them without therapy.

Sometimes effective therapy is self-therapy, and therapy is always better than no therapy; no former addict has ever recovered without continuing support. Some popular actors, singers, politicians, athletes and models who have been known for their distractive lifestyle, and who had persistent problems with alcohol and drugs, were under pressure to cure themselves alone.

Learning to control the use of alcohol and drugs is not simple. Such control requires a high level of self awareness: a capacity that is almost invariably diminished by substances. Few users remain capable to honest self-scrutiny to sustain control. Most regular-to-heavy drug users lie to their bosses, to their spouses, to their friends and lovers, and lie to themselves. By the time most users are ready to quit, drug taking has become too consuming and threatening to their lives.

Once an individual becomes physically dependent, drugs serve as secondary reinforcers, in that they function to relieve real or anticipated abstinence symptoms. Wikler's theory[58] postulates that most attempts to reduce pain pharmacologically are classically conditioned. The addict becomes conditioned to the drug. Exposure to stimuli or cues associated with previous episodes of opiate self-administration and/or withdrawal constitutes an obstacle for relapse. Stimuli such as "shooting up" or being in an environment or culture in which drugs were previously consumed, in combination with internal cues (feeling tense, depressed, or bored) can trigger an increase in drug craving which is then followed by drug-seeking behavior.

According to the National Survey on Drug Use and Health,[59] about 18.3 million persons ages 12 or older are classified with alcohol dependency or abuse. According to Wayne Buckwalter, families often do not know what to do, what therapy to choose or what is available to them, and as a result do nothing, which is harmful to recovering addicts who need a strong support system. Recovery is a day to day battle. Certain people, places and things could serve as triggers for relapse. Even after treatment, the path to recovery is filled with obstacles.

Effective therapy requires a high level of disclosure and confidentiality. Privacy means controlling access to information. Confidentiality means controlling how private information is handled, managed, and disseminated. Confidentiality is assumed in a therapeutic relationship unless prior warning is given. There is implicit promise and trust; there is respect for autonomy in caring for the treated individuals; there is disposition towards honoring personal wishes and maintaining intimate details of personal lives confidential.

The therapist is unlikely to get involved in insight therapies during an outpatient drug treatment. Topics of interest for those in an outpatient program may be: social adjustment, relationships with family and friends, difficulties at school or on the job, and the setting of treatment goals. Treatment is more effective if it demands regular, frequent participation in group counseling. Those that are part of a larger mental health system, or favor traditional mental health practices, give counseling

---

[58] Wikler's Theory (1965, 1968). Psychological and behavioral techniques in managing pain. PubMed.

[59] Substance Abuse and Mental Health Services Administration (2012). National Survey on Drug Use and Health.

more weight than group therapy. Individuals find support for new behavior in the group, opportunities to share experiences, discover new insights and create goals, and come up with ways to assess progress toward abstinence.

Patients are much more likely to benefit from therapy despite the fact that there may be an inordinate resistance in a group setting. Group members have no control over how their disclosures are being used and therefore are reluctant to carry out meaningful group therapy, especially in outpatient programs. Another issue that has been problematic is the tendency of some groups using group pressure to accomplish dubious goals.

Support

Finding Meaning in Life

The third step in quitting addiction is establishing support. The rewarding effects of drugs and alcohol, which drive an individual to drink and use drugs again, result in the absence of any better rewards for staying sober. Rewards could only come by accepting suffering as an inescapable part of the transformation we call recovery. To achieve recovery and adhere to abstinence, individuals with addiction have to act on difficult choices and make sacrifices. Making sacrifices means suffering and suffering forces that individual to ask what his/her suffering is for and what it means.

Suffering triggers the urge to escape and without meaning there is not an enduring reason to stay sober. Spiritual growth begins with faith, hope and love. An addict can realize this by looking at the drink and seeing how he lost his job, family and health. One day the wife, the children, the boss and clients may show love and appreciation, but the next they may not. If an addict counts on others' constant affection and admiration, s/he is likely to be disappointed.

More help persists from recovering alcoholics and the addicts themselves, sharing their strength, hope, and experience. It cannot be found on TV and the Internet; the TV and Internet are simulations used to escape from loneliness, boredom and fear. If the relief offered by drugs and alcohol is not replaced by better and reliable rewards, then the addict, who is trying to abstain, feels trapped and resentful. Recovery is work, and points to something beyond the self (and not all aspects of growth are bright).[60]

Attending to the present moment of consciousness requires effort and learning to live in it demands unending effort. Many addicts do not realize this effort is needed, since little things become trivial to their lives. Some behaviors that would have been unacceptable become tolerable. They tell themselves countless excuses,

---

[60]   Sandor, R. (2009). *Thinking Simply About Addiction.* London: Penguin Books.

rationalize and convince themselves that nothing was wrong. They do not have to deal with the present and their feelings; the drugs make all the hardships "disappear". Drugs help combat boredom, isolation and loneliness. The longer drugs are used, the more distorted the perception and judgment became. Drugs turned out to be the focus and meaning of life, and social connections are not made over the drugs.

Recovering drug addicts are instrumental for addicts who are trying to find new meaning in life. They inquire why the addicted individuals feel bored, rejected, or unattractive. Former addicts can help addict find what to do to improve their life by filling it with hobbies and personal pursuits instead of drugs. Being productive is a way that clearly benefits the addicts and is associated with finding meaning and an improved self-esteem.

The immediate consequences of stopping using drugs may be: emptiness, overwhelming feelings, inability to study or work, gaining weight, and disappointing sex. Healthy alternatives involve calm surroundings, meditating in a quiet place and participating in outdoor recreation activities. Breathing techniques and yoga are a great complementary treatment which help relieve anxiety due to the amount of oxygen and carbon dioxide that the body accumulates during these activities. The vagus nerve, which is excited during these activities, connects to several parts of the brain, including certain fibers in the thalamus that decreases activity in the frontal cortex and lower anxiety. The hypothalamus improves alertness and attention, and produces feelings of satisfaction and pleasure. Addicts must change their perception that drugs are the only answer to boosting self-esteem and improving mood.

Stimulants such as crystal meth and cocaine pump up feelings of self-worth, allowing users a temporary sense of confidence, power and self-acceptance. Quiet individuals feel happy, and start to be talkative, engaging, attractive, and desirable. While the drug makes the brain think happy, researchers have found that one of the strongest determinants of happiness is having a meaningful life and interpersonal relations which are usually lost when people become severely addicted. Former addicts are an excellent support resource. They are emphatic but can also be confronting when needed. Confrontation however might be uncomfortable, and if the addict is defensive, it can seem offensive. The addict hides from the problem by escaping with drugs and avoiding the problem, which leads to growing feelings of powerlessness and hopelessness. Alcohol or heroin make people care less and feel numb to disappointment. Coming to terms with their addiction and short falls brings awareness. Addicts must have awareness into their own likes, dislikes, and vulnerabilities to get out of stressful situations. They cannot set irrational or unrealistic expectations but they can become aware of unconscious desires.

Friends who do drugs know how to target someone's vulnerabilities, and the dealers want to make money. It is not uncommon to give away free drugs in an attempt to gain back customers. The recovered addict must exercise saying no thanks ("I am taking a break") to the "free" drugs. Moving to a new place and making changes to the environment are often part of recovery. Sticking to a structured schedule is also a basic principle in finding meaning. Keeping the mind occupied and engaged in community service projects or in self-relaxation techniques increases the likelihood that the addict would be sober at any time.

It is essential for addicts to make contact with significant others and at the same time compose a personal list of old friends to avoid. If they cannot completely be avoided, they must plan what to say and do in each one of these situations. Or the recovered addict needs to let those contacts go and move on. When a person becomes an addict, the order of his/her priorities changes; his/her health, family career, and work suffer. As part of a drug culture users make a common bond, and at that time it seems there is no one to replace that bond. American culture views addiction as a weakness of character. It blames the individual for being an addict, and the shame makes it even harder for the addict to admit to having a problem and seek help. The individual's self perception has a tremendous effect on his/her recovery. Biological and organic depression can add to the distress and may cause social withdrawal, feelings of hopelessness, low energy, and poor motivation. All of which can keep the recovering addict stuck in a rut that prevents him/her from finding new meaning in life, and puts him/her at risk for relapse.

Yoga has been suggested by eastern spiritual leaders as an activity of meaning that focuses on the here-and-now, looks at the present moment in time and brings peace and meaning to the mind. Yoga is particularly helpful with patients who suffer from depression without taking conventional antidepressant medications. Those with any serious medical illness should consult their physicians before considering a yoga program. This includes women who are pregnant, or those with medical conditions such as uncontrolled high blood pressure, seizure disorders, significant heart disease, or who have had recent injuries or surgery. Also, bipolar disorders with psychotic symptoms may be worsened.

Meditation is another way to achieve a meaningful state from within the mind, and massage complements this by physically forcing a relaxed state from within the body. Holding hands near the addict's body without any actual physical contact (Reiki) is a form that acts as a conduit to direct the energy back into the addict. Reiki is an alternative for minimal to no physical contact. Yoga, meditation, massage, and Reiki therapies bring us closer to earth in order to connect with our roots and find meaning. They create positive energy and vitality.

In a social experiment, a designated individual refuses all drugs for two weeks while the others were free to use them. The attention of the experiment was on what happened among the group members of the drug culture. As an outside observer, this individual learned important things about him/herself and his/her "friends". Friends who put him/her at risk were not real friends. This kind of reaction forced him to look for meaning in life. His defensive mechanisms brought him bank the most familiar maladaptive coping strategy which was the drug.

Unfortunately, there is a culture to drug use; drugs are likely to be the glue that holds much of the drug "doing" group to stick together. Addicts should look for friends who like them for who they are and not because they do drugs together and party. Some individuals think they need to have friends who use drugs with them to make their own drug use more acceptable; they are helping themselves feel less guilty about their own drug use.

References

1. *Deseret News*, September 2, 2012.
2. *Deseret News*, September 16, 2012.
3. *Brain in the News*, October 2011.
4. *Deseret News*, August 5, 2012.
5. Khantzian, E. J., & Albense, M. J. (2008) Understanding Addiction as Self Medication: Finding Hope Behind the Pain. Lanham, MD: Rowman & Littlefield.
6. Khantzian, E. J., & Albense, M. J. (2008, p. 109).
7. Lee, S. (2006). Becoming Crystal Meth Addiction. New York: Marlow & Company.
8. *Time Magazine*, September, 2010.
9. Bernard, S. (2010, Dec. 1). Neuro myths: Separating fact and fiction in brain based learning. *Brain in the News*, pp. 2-3.
10. Thakkar, V. G., Collins, C, & Levitt, P. (2006). Addiction. New York: Chelsea House.
11. Gunderson, E. W. (2011, December). Buprenorphine induction: A major barrier for physician adoption of office-based opioid dependence treatment. *Journal of Addiction Medicine*, 5(4), 304-305.
12. Mirin, S. M. (1984). Substance Abuse and Psychopathology. Washington D.C.: American Psychiatric Press.
13. Williams, J. S. *NIDA Notes*, Vol. 18(5), pp.1-4.
14. Health Services (2012, April 08) Princeton, NJ: Princeton University, p. 71.

15. Health Services (2012, April 08) Princeton, NJ: Princeton University, p. 72.
16. Brain glutamate concentration affects cocaine seeking. *NIDA Notes*, Vol. 19, pp. 3.
17. NIDA Notes, vol 20(5), pp. 8-10.
18. Whitten, L. Community-based treatment benefits methamphetamine abusers. *NIDA Notes*, Vol. 20(5), pp. 4-6.
19. Zickler, P. Brain activity patterns signal risk of relapse to methamphetamines. *NIDA Notes*, Vol. 20(5), pp. 1-3.
20. Zickler, P. Network therapy expands treatment capabilities of small practice providers. *NIDA Notes*: Research findings. Vol. 18, No. 2, pp. 5-7.
21. *Salt Lake City Tribune*, April 3, 2011, pp. 1, 6.
22. Farrer, S. Alternative cigarettes may deliver more nicotine then conventional cigarettes. *NIDA Notes*. Vol 18, No 2, pp. 8-9.
23. Hans, S. (1978). The Stress of Life. New York: McGraw-Hill.
24. *NIDA Notes*. Vol 18, No. 5. pp. 1-3.
25. New technology expands the scope of NIDA's intramural Brain imaging program. *NIDA Notes*. Vol 18, No. 2, pp. 14-15
26. *Brain in the News*, October 2011.
27. Animal experiments in addiction science. *NIDA Notes*. Vol 20(5). pp. 11-18.
28. Animal research shows GHB acts on GABA receptors. *NIDA Notes*. Vol 20(5).
29. Williams, J. S. (n.d.) Early use of drugs may lead to later psychiatric disorders. *NIDA Notes*. Vol 18(5), pp. 1-2.
30. Henderson, E. C. (2000). Understanding Addiction. University Press of Mississippi.
31. *Brain in the News*, December 2010.
32. Substance Abuse and Mental Health Services Administration (2012). Drug addiction: The emotional life (p. 126)
33. Relationships matter: Impact of parental, peer factors on teen, young adult substance abuse. *NIDA Notes*, Vol 18, No. 2
34. DeLa Rosa, M., Holleran, L., & Straussner, S. L. A. (2005). Substance-Abusing Latinos. New York: Haworth Press.
35. Denizet-Lewis, B. (2009). America Anonymous. New York: Simon & Schuster.
36. Jung, C. G. (1981). The Archetypes and the Collective Unconscious. Collected Works of C. G. Jung, Vol. 9 Part 1. New Jersey: Princeton University Press.
37. Cozolino, L. (2006). The Neuroscience of Human Relationships: Attachment and the Developing Social Brain. New York: WW Norton & Company.
38. Dispenza, J. (2009). The Science of Changing the Mind. Health Communications, Incorporated.
39. Meichenbaum, D. (1995). A Clinical Handbook/Practical Therapist Manual for Assessing and Treating Adults with Post-Traumatic Stress Disorder (PTSD).

Waterloo, Ontario, Canada: Institute Press: Donald Meichenbaum, University of Waterloo.

40. Nietzsche, F. (1954). The Portable Nietzsche. (Walter Kaufmann, Trans.) New York: Penguin.
41. Deleuze, G. (2006) [1983], Nietzsche and Philosophy. (Hugh Tomlinson, trans.). Athlone Press.
42. Keller, H. (1996). The Story of My Life. Dover. Mineola, NY.
43. *Deseret News*, September 21, 2012.
44. Lieberman, A. F., Van Horn P, & Ozer E. (2005). The impact of domestic violence on preschoolers: Predictive and mediating factors. *Development and Psychopathology*, 17(2), 385-96.
45. Cozolino, L. (2006). The Neuroscience of Human Relationships. New York: Norton and Company.
46. Lieberman, A. F. & Van Horn, P. (2005).Toward evidence-based treatment. *Journal of American Academy of Child Adolescence Psychiatry*, 44(12).
47. Marohn, S. (2003) The Natural Medicine Guide to Addiction. Charlottesville, Va. Hampton Roads.
48. Deseret News, August 5, 2012.
49. Parade, June 12, 2011.
50. Finnigan, C. (2008) When Enough is Enough. New York: Penguin Group.
51. Gwinnell, E. (2006). The A to Z of Addiction and Addictive Behaviors. New York.
52. Deseret News, January 6, 2013.
53. Deseret News, August 5, 2012.
54. Brain in the News, May 2012.
55. Khantzlan, E. J., & Albanese, M. J. (2008)
56. Brain in the News, October, 2011.
57. Stuart, L. (1972) Cognitive Behavior Therapy. Hoboken, NJ: Wiley
58. Wikler's Theory (1965, 1968). Psychological and behavioral techniques in managing pain. PubMed.
59. Substance Abuse and Mental Health Services Administration (2012). National Survey on Drug Use and Health.
60. Sandor, R. (2009). Thinking Simply About Addiction. London: Penguin Books.

Appendix A

GREENSPAN DEVELOPMENTAL MODEL has six stages in the development of a child:

Stage 1: Security: The ability to look, listen, and be calm–the first developmental skill is the ability to be calm and regulated and at the same time be interested and engaged in the world.

Stage 2: Relating: The Ability to Feel Warm and Close to Others–children with special needs, particularly those with obvious physical or psychological abnormalities, are at increased risk for problems at this stage because of how cruel other kids can be. When a child expects to be humiliated or teased because of how he looks or acts, the best (and natural) defense is to isolate and avoid other kids. Because most learning occurs in the context of relationships, avoiding others results in significant problems with all later stages of development.

Stage 3: Intentional: Two-Way Communication without Words–developing the capacity to focus and relate to others allows children to begin communicating with willful intention through facial expressions, gestures, and body language. By 18 months of age, many children are quite good at reading nonverbal cues and engaging in the most rudimentary forms of communication. It is through learning to read nonverbal language in others that we learn to differentiate emotions in other people, and how to send and receive nonverbal messages that establish our personal boundaries. For children who grow-up in families where parents are not well equipped to facilitate emotional growth (because they are stuck developmentally themselves), academic success can become the primary vehicle for a child's sense of self, leading to advanced degrees and professional careers where intelligence is highly valued. For many who follow such a path, the price of academic and professional success comes at a significant cost-developmental constrictions and deficits in reading nonverbal cues, subtle emotional gestures, and knowing how to deeply engage with all sorts of people in different contexts.

Stage 4: Solving Problems and Forming a Sense of Self-children begin to solve problems with the help of others.

Stage 5: Emotional Ideas–children (and many adults) who never fully master the skills of this stage, have difficulty identifying what they are feeling and instead simply act-out feelings in actions and behaviors. Many who drink excessively or use illicit drugs do so in response to feelings that are difficult to identify, talk about, and experience (therapist offer parents' emotion coaching).

Stage 6: Emotional Thinking–the capacity the one has to reflect on future behavior, feel empathy for others, and realize that actions can have consequences, require mastery of the skills of emotional thinking.

ABOUT THE AUTHOR

"I have known Dr. Merav Nagel for more than 10 years. Throughout those years, I have observed a rare and undiminished passion to childhood education, specifically children with learning disabilities. Her two PhD's, post-doctoral fellowships, and the many publications she authored are a small testimony to the breadth and depth of her expertise ranging from various learning disabilities like dyslexia and attention deficit disorder to sports psychology, emotional eating, substance abuse, and stress management. She connects the dots between the biological functions, emotional states and learning challenges sprinkling a wealth of experience and wisdom along the way. I strongly support and recommend Dr. Nagel's work. I look forward to someday collaborating with Dr. Nagel in spreading the kind of knowledge educators and parents starve from knowing in their efforts to serve as the pillars for the generations to come."

Dr. Patrick G Mauroy, Atlanta GA

ABOUT THE EDITOR

Nicole Fisher graduated from Westminster College of Salt Lake City, Utah, the department of Science in Psychology. She was involved in many research projects and completed a thesis on risk and self-disclosure. She is continuing her graduate studies with the department of psychology at the University of Utah. Fisher intends to become an independent researcher and a teacher.

www.ingramcontent.com/pod-product-compliance
Lightning Source LLC
Chambersburg PA
CBHW022002170526
45157CB00003B/1108